25 REASONS
WHY WE MUST BE
OUR OWN DOCTOR

How Being Our Own Doctor Can Help
Us Stay Healthier, Gain Self Respect And
Keep Money In Our Pocket.

Pieter Rijke, BScPT, LLM

<u>**25 Reasons Why We Must Be Our Own Doctor**</u>

ISBN 978-0-9939676-0-3

First Printing November 2014

Published in Canada by Pieter Rijke
www.westbankpublishing.com

Table of Contents

The Secret Of Proper Health Care Is Giving The Patient What He Wants

About the author

Pieter is originally from the Netherlands, where he studied physiotherapy, Traditional Chinese Medicine and law.
He worked as a physiotherapist and acupuncturist in the Netherlands and Germany, before he immigrated with his family to British Columbia, Canada in 1999. He worked in Canada in hospitals and set up several physiotherapy clinics. He owned an acupuncture clinic in Kelowna, BC, for 6 years.
Pieter worked on cruise ships during a couple of years as an acupuncturist, where he treated patients from all over the world.
His international background gives him a unique opportunity to mold a view on health and health care, based on his experiences with so many different cultures.
Pieter continues to work as a physiotherapist and acupuncturist in British Columbia, where he applies his views on proper health care and motivates his patients to take control over their health as much as possible.

Acknowledgements

I want to thank my wife Brigitte for always having believed in me and for being the stimulating force to finally get these words on paper and out there for people to read.

I also want to thank Jeff McCallum, co-author of '101 Reasons Why You Must Write A Book'. After reading his book I was finally ready to finish mine.

I want to thank my daughters Annabelle and Claire for unconditional support and friends and family who gave valuable advice.

Introduction

I have been involved in health care since 1979, as a physical therapist and acupuncturist in different settings and in different countries. I did other things in my life, like working for a big commercial bank and getting a law degree, but eventually I stayed in health care. I owned several private clinics, I worked in hospitals and care homes and on cruise ships. I have practised in The Netherlands, where I was born, in Germany, in Canada, where I live now and I treated patients from all nationalities on a three year cruise ship adventure, from Alaska to The Caribbean and across the Atlantic to the Mediterranean.
Of course when I started I treated everybody according to the book, using the rules I learned during my study. I was enthusiastic and had good results, not always, but enough to keep me going.
As soon as I finished my physiotherapy study in the Netherlands I decided to get a degree in Traditional Chinese Medicine, because that had always interested me.
Both studies are working according to certain rules; in that respect there is no difference between east and west. So again, after completing Chinese medicine, I happily and enthusiastically applied what I had learned in my clinic. I had good results, not always, but enough to keep me going.
After a couple of years I started to feel moments of frustration, because there were quite some situations where I could not get results or the problems went away but came back again.

I knew of course that it is impossible to always get good results, but I felt that there was more that could be done, but it just hadn't taken shape yet. What was health care supposed to do for people, in a gentle and effective way, worthy of a human being?

Eventually I needed all those thirty-plus years to find an answer for myself. And I needed the insights from modern medicine as well as those from ancient medicine to mold and shape it.

It is still difficult to put it down in words, but I have a clearer picture now.

This is not a book about all kinds of alternative remedies for different ailments; if that is what you want to know, you can go online and read forever. It is a book about making people conscious about whom they are, what they can accomplish and how they can fight to maintain their self-value, especially when it comes to health care. Too often are we sucked into the system and being treated with protocols, by professionals, who are not really interested in our wellbeing and are not listening to us. If I talk about doctors, I don't just mean physicians, but all health care professionals.

This is the goal of my book: to deliver a message to patients everywhere, of all categories, about health, how to get it and maintain it and, above all, how to maintain your self-esteem. There is a plethora of authors, who have done the same thing, but it all comes from the heart and all those hearts are different.

I hope you will like my heart.

*Our Medical System Is Based On The Same Principles
And Works Within The Same Circumstances
As Those That Make Us Sick In The First Place*

Chapter 1

What is healthcare?

The last thing I want is to give the impression that I am against modern medicine, because I am not. It has tremendous potential and is essential in lifesaving, acute care. I just want to give it the place it deserves, nothing more, nothing less.

When we think about healthcare, we think about hospitals, care homes, doctors, nurses, medication and so on; big institutions that swallow money for food and are intimidating and commanding. They are distant and we try hard to stay away from them, because once in it is difficult to get out. Once in, they take our personality away, our capacity to make decisions, our opinion. We are not heard; we have to follow the yellow line and wait, wait. There is no individuality, no time and not always compassion. Health care, the care for our physical and emotional wellbeing, the most personal thing there is, has become a model of impersonality.
And we, as patients, let it all happen. We have slowly manoeuvred ourselves in this position, and if we don't change, nothing will change.

What does the dictionary say about healthcare? Just the first one that I found online:

...the prevention, treatment, and management of illness and t he preservation of mental and physical wellbeing through the services offered by the medical and allied health professions.[1]

This definition assumes that one can only become healthy through intervention of a third person or institution. In other words, health care, the ultimate form of personality, is not in our hands, but in somebody else's.

Let's try another one, randomly:

Health care (or healthcare) is the diagnosis, treatment, and prevention of disease, illness, injury, and other physical and mental impairments in humans. Health care is delivered by practitioners in medicine, optometry, dentistry, nursing, pharmacy, allied health, and other care providers. It refers to the work done in providing primary care, secondary care and tertiary care, as well as in public health.[2]

Again, third persons are delivering the care, not us.

This is not about Stedman's Medical Dictionary or Wikipedia, but about the general, public perception of what health care is, obviously not something that especially involves us, but mainly others, the providers. Some

---

[1] health care. (n.d.). *The American Heritage® Stedman's Medical Dictionary.* Retrieved May 28, 2013, from Dictionary.com website:http://dictionary.reference.com/browse/health care
[2] Wikipedia

definitions even just mention social insurance as a payment option and don't talk about patients at all.

I also found this one:

1. ...the field concerned with the maintenance or restoration of the health of the body or mind.
2. any of the procedures or methods employed in this field.[3]

This is, of course, much closer to what it should be. This is what healthcare is and now we can start thinking about who should be delivering it.

Human beings are basically very simple. We all have certain basic needs and desires that need to be fulfilled: the need to eat, to have sex, to be respected and appreciated, the need to survive. If we find this, we are happy and at ease, if we do not, we become unbalanced and are prone to dis-ease. We spend most of our life looking for ways to satisfy these needs, because if we manage to do so, we confirm our individuality, and that is what it is all about. We buy a big house so that we can eat in it and have sex in it, but also because we want to show people that we can afford it, so they will respect us. We will throw parties in it so we will be appreciated and we will feel our individuality grow. Give a derailed person an important task to do and tell him that only he can do it and very shortly he will be back on track again, because we have recognised his individuality.
It is very difficult in this hectic society to get recognition and confirmation of who we are. Society is not really interested in individuals, there are too many of us, like ants: you cannot tell them apart. But that does not mean that we

---

[3] healthcare. (n.d.). *Dictionary.com Unabridged*. Retrieved May 28, 2013, from Dictionary.com website: http://dictionary.reference.com/browse/healthcare

don't feel the need to be recognised. People will go to great lengths to find confirmation and if nothing works they become criminal. That is another way of getting attention.

This constant fight in search for our personality is tiring and exhausting. It is very stressful and demanding and burns our energy away. And because of the complexity of this world we really have to do our utmost to stick out above the rest, to be noticed. Many people will not succeed and give up and they can easily become depressed, because we are not judged by who we are, but by what we accomplish.

Our bodies and minds are perfect organisms, created to survive under many circumstances. For example, when danger threatens we produce stress hormones, like cortisol and adrenaline. Cortisol releases sugars in the bloodstream, so that we can generate more energy and adrenaline raises the blood pressure, speeds up the heart rate and makes us alert. So, in days gone by, when we woke up in the morning and found a huge cave bear at the entrance of our dwelling, we would have all the ingredients prepared to run for our lives and in the process of doing so we would burn away the stress hormones and in the end we would be at peace again (if we ran fast enough, that is). So the body and mind would be in balance again and hopefully that bear encounter would not happen every day.
Back to the present: we wake up in the morning, shower and dress and go to work. We have to participate in traffic, somebody runs a red light or gives us the finger, no parking place, late for work and so on. Each of those occurrences probably produces the same amount of stress hormones as the adventure with the cave bear and it is only 8.30 AM. Plus, we don`t really do anything with the energy boost and elevated heart rate and blood pressure. So the stress

hormones are sitting there, unused, and become toxic to the body. Liver, kidneys and all the filters and systems we have to clean rubbish out of our body, are starting to sweep and clean. Probably, they were still working on the results of yesterday, and therefore easily become overworked. This goes on and on, everyday. The body cannot handle it anymore and opens the door for sickness, like allergies, kidney failure, skin conditions, because the toxins have to go somewhere. There is no balance, no basis for health. If you read about longevity, people that become far over a hundred years old, like 120 and more, are always living in remote areas, on higher elevations with fresh air, who eat what the land provides, who perform hard physical labour their whole lives and who have a minimum of stress. They know the land, the people, the weather and what is expected from them. They are in balance with themselves and their surroundings.

This process of getting sick is all based on overload. Too much input for body and mind. We are not made to handle all that and our bodies give us warning upon warning, but it is very hard to listen and often hard to change. **Our medical system is also not helping, because it is based on the same principles and works within the same circumstances as those that make us sick in the first place.** Our body and mind are looking for rest and balance, the only way to get better, but are we finding that in the waiting rooms of doctors and hospitals? How can a body that has been battered over and over again with overuse, toxic material, stress and so on, get better by a drug (toxic in itself) administered by a health care practitioner who does not have time for our problem and might not even be interested? How can surgery, North America's beloved panacea after drugs, solve a problem that started in the first place because of a lack of balance, by creating even more imbalance in the body?

This morning there was an announcement on the news, about a new drug for prostate cancer. It was promising and offered hope for men suffering from this affliction. If I would have prostate cancer in a late stage without much hope, I would probably be first in line for this drug, but at the same time I would wonder what it would really do for me, and what I could expect from it in the long run. What would the side effects be, how would it affect my immune system and energy level, and, most important of all, how would it involve me in the healing process?

What I want to say with this story about health care is that it is about our health, not the doctor's. We have the first responsibility. We cannot all live in remote areas on high elevations, or be hermits and stare at our belly buttons all day, sitting cross-legged on a mountaintop, but there is a lot we can do.

So first we need to realize that health care is not administered by others, but by us. Health care is not the administration of something after we become sick, but it is our way of living, it is prevention and making sure we are in balance.

Summary

Healthcare is not what others provide for us, but what we provide for ourselves. We have needs and desires and are constantly busy satisfying them. That is difficult, because society is not really interested in our individuality, so we easily get sick. Our body reacts in a logical way to the circumstances we are in, but if the circumstances are not logical, but chaotic, our body's reaction can make us sick, due to overload and too much input. Our mainstream medical system does not help, because it is based on the same values that make us sick. We need to look for responsibility, prevention and balance.

Sickness Is Dis-ease

Chapter 2

Sickness

The way people look at sickness depends a lot on their culture and background. Simpler living communities, who don't have so many goods and possessions, and therefore less stress, accept a lot of discomfort as part of life, things that for us would be a reason to go to the doctor. Think about menopause, a normal process the female body has to go through, yet a reason to visit the doctor and request medication (hormonal) in many places and by doing so introducing new toxic material to an otherwise healthy system.
Another example is allergies. During the winter our body collects all kinds of toxic material, we eat more and heavier and usually move less. In the spring, the time of great clean-up, our body wants to get rid of all that and tries to do that through coughing, sneezing, watery eyes and so on. That is, in fact, a perfectly healthy process, but, for us it is very inconvenient, so we suppress this reaction with medication. Medication is toxic and in the end makes it all worse.
Think about all the things we do to slow down aging, like using all kinds of cosmetics, Botox injections and surgeries. Believe me, no matter how innocent they say this all is, it is not, because it is an attack on the integrity of our body. And why would we want to slow down aging in the first place? The reason must be that we don't accept death as a part of

life anymore. Life and death are in balance, but balance is a concept that has lost its value nowadays.

One of the greatest dangers to our health is inflammation. It turns out that almost all forms of sickness begin with inflammation. I am not talking about the inflammation we can clearly see and feel, like an infected finger or the effects of an insect bite, I mean chronic inflammation that exists inside our body and festers year after year.

Whenever we are injured the body's first response is to fix it. It does this by mobilizing chemicals to clean and heal and send them to the affected area. Think about white blood cells, endorphins, muscle relaxants, whatever is needed to heal the problem as fast as possible. The problem is that our body does this every time when it receives a signal that something is wrong, and something is wrong continuously in our modern day life. There are so many stress factors attacking our body on a daily basis, like loud noises, bright lights, fights, traffic, hurry, pressure, air pollution, food, drinks, drugs, expectations that cannot be fulfilled and the list goes on. It is a constant bombardment of stressors that brings our body in a constant state of alertness and therefore in a constant state of inflammation.

It is now believed that cardiovascular diseases like stroke and heart attack can be the result of chronic inflammation in the blood vessels. Inflammation is also believed to be involved in the start of neurological diseases like Parkinson and MS and for the widespread existence of diabetes, depression and cancer.

Inflammation is inherently warm. In Traditional Chinese Medicine this would be called yang. So our body is carrying too much yang inside and we need to balance that with yin, the opposite. Almost everything in modern life is yang, too hot and hyper. It is like we forgot how to bring rest and relaxation in our life (yin) and therefore we get all these hyper forms of disease.

Summary

Sickness is culturally determined. What we see as sickness, others will see as a natural reaction of the body to certain circumstances. In our modern world we have too many factors working on our health and disturbing it.

We Can't See The Patient For The Trees

Chapter 3

Modern Lifestyle

I think we can easily say that modern life is complex, stressful and demanding, just to name a few topics. There is no simplicity anymore, no norms and values that we can take for granted, as we did for so long in the past. I like to believe that with my 63 years I am not very old, but when I think back of my childhood the differences are enormous. Everything that seemed holy and untouchable for us in those days is now for the grab. I think for example of sexuality, politeness, responsibility, respect, manners, use of violence, social pressure, egocentrism and so on. People are becoming more and more isolated from the world and others. Looking around us we only see people lost in their cellphones and wearing earphones, not really participating in life. I call it degeneration signs. At the end of every civilisation comes a time of moral decline. People have too many goods and possessions, too much money. The same thing happened at the end of the Roman Empire, with the likes of Emperor Caligula and Nero, or in modern China, after the suffocating grip of communism and the opening of their market to the West.
It makes people weak and prone to sickness and addictions. We can easily become addicted to almost anything, be it drugs, nicotine, alcohol, food, sex or, in short, to anything

that makes us feel good. We even become addicted to our own endorphins. Endorphins are chemicals the brain produces, also called 'feel good hormones'. They are extremely strong painkillers, many times stronger than morphine. We produce these endorphins as a reaction to stress (positive or negative), pain and fear. Why are people running a marathon? That is 40 kilometers of torture for the body, but the rewards are the production of lots of endorphins. So it makes us feel good and it allows us to finish the job. The more endorphins it produces, the more we want to run, or workout, or have sex or smoke or do whatever else makes us feel good.

So that is the reason that everybody is frequenting the gym these days. I worked on cruise ships for a couple of years and these ships have huge gyms, with all possible equipment. On embarkation day, about two hours after it started, the gym was packed, 30 treadmills all taken, 20 stationary bikes, lots of steppers, elliptical trainers, stair climbers and rows of sweating, often overweight people working with weights. I often stood there and looked at it and thought: this cannot be right.

And it is not right. People with sitting and stressful jobs should not workout like there is no tomorrow, as soon as vacation begins. But the same goes for more experienced and well-trained athletes. There is more and more scientific evidence that marathons, for example, are creating inflammation in the body, increasing the risk of heart attack and stroke, even for professional runners. And the same thing is valid for other high activity sports. The reason is simple: nothing in the body works abrupt, with spurts of energy. The body wants to assimilate and take time to adjust to new circumstances; then it maintains balance in the nervous system and that makes us feel good.

Without endorphins we would not like to run or exhaust our self. There are also activities that we like anyway, without overproduction of endorphins, for example going to a party. But even that can take a lot of energy away from the body, if we don't do it in a wise way. The problem is that it is very hard to know ones limits.

The good thing is that our body will always let us know in what state it is, what it can do and cannot do. If we learn how to listen and recognize signs and messages, we can anticipate and be active in a responsible way. Doing that means that we have to concentrate on our self, on what is going on in *our* body and *our* mind. We have to say goodbye to what society says and science, to what the doctor says and what our friends say, because the answer to our questions is deep inside our self. If we just know how to listen.

If you think that that is very difficult, a good starting point is meditation. I don't know how it is with you, but when I first heard the word meditation, in the 60-ties, it was all psychedelic and surrounded by flower power and Bhagwan followers. It still has that ring to it a little bit, but we know now a lot more about the benefits of meditation. The earlier forms of meditation are all from oriental origin, like transcendental meditation and several yoga techniques. They are very effective, but there are big differences between us Westerners and Orientals, especially when it comes to things of the mind. More and more meditation techniques have been developed overtime by Westerners, like Progressive Muscle Relaxation, Autogenic Training and forms of self-hypnosis. These techniques are more focused on the Western consumer and use a very straightforward concept.

With Progressive Muscle Relaxation, for example, we focus on muscle tension and try to release that by concentration. Autogenic Training is a more complete relaxation technique that concentrates on 6 basic functions of the body: muscle activity, blood circulation, breathing, nervous system, heart function and brain control. A German psychologist developed it and it is focused on things that we can feel and be aware of. The first exercise concentrates on our muscles and the feeling of heaviness, the second on warmth, as a direct result of the relaxation of our muscles. There are 4 more exercises, all depending on each other. The beauty of this system is that we can teach our self in about two months to relax in almost any given circumstance.

But it is not necessary to follow a pre-cooked system; we can definitely develop our own way of meditation. What we want to do is try to empty our mind for a short while and experience the sensation of being absolutely worry-free. During that time our body is completely in balance and all systems function the way they should. It is also a state that can make us aware of what is wrong in our body. A good example of this is this: if we have an injury, let us say a shoulder pain, and we relax for a while, most of the time our shoulder pain gets worse in the beginning. The reason is that it is much harder to relax the muscles around the injured shoulder, because they are performing a protective action. Automatically we become aware of the problem, when we are able to dim the rest of the lights.

Instead of spending all those hours on physical workouts it would be so much more effective if we integrated half an hour of meditation in our daily schedule. Then, the physical body works better without having to torture it with too much exercise. Too much exercise is in fact a stressful thing for us and can threaten our body overtime.

But, because we are human beings, we like to behave like the rest of us. We like to follow the rules society imposes on us. So, if society is of the opinion that we need to workout a lot in order to be 'healthy', we just want to comply. Society has so many rules: we want to look good and stay young, to make money, to be successful. We also want to be appreciated and admired. And we definitely do not accept death as part of our life. In order to do all that we need to do things that are not healthy. Taking Botox injections to look good and stay young is not healthy, whatever they want you to believe. It is still a (toxic) product that does not belong in the body. Facelifts are surgical procedures that drain energy and leave scar tissue. Making money and being successful requires long hours of work, social deprivation and a lot of stress. Eventually this kind of life leads to addiction, because people like having money, like feeling the thrill of a good business deal, and last but not least the satisfaction of having status. And we want more and more. The need for appreciation and admiration, two of our basic needs to survive, comes with a price. And don't we know it: everybody recognises the feeling of frustration, exhaustion and emptiness while participating in the rat race. But the alternative is a feeling of shortcoming, failure and unhappiness. Not participating makes us feel like a loser. The question is of course if that is right: how can we be a loser if we decide to follow our own way and make our own choices? I admire people who make daring decisions, who go into the opposite direction and take risks. Who give up a good paying job, with securities and benefits, just to live a quiet live, away from stress. I sometimes think that they are the only ones who really understand the value of life.

The struggle to keep up with the demands of modern day life is a reason for many of us to develop sickness. Depression is a good example. Depression becomes more and more widespread and it is a typical example of what can happen to body and mind if we don't take time for our self. Many young people, like teenagers, cannot handle the combined pressure of growing up and trying to keep up with society and its expectations and choose to leave this life, before it even begins. For a teenager, stepping out of the circle of peers would be a disaster and he would immediately be stigmatized.

Our society is no longer focused on balance. It cannot get a grip. When the complexity of life becomes too strong it tries to douse the flames and treat the symptoms, because the alternative, drastically change our lifestyle, is too threatening and risky. **So, choosing for our self is too risky, think about that**. It means that we continue to become sick and unbalanced and let the cancer grow. How risky is that? The more we participate in the rules of society the faster the cancer grows. The modern answer, to treat with –long term- medication will not solve the problem, because it creates new ones at the same time.

Lots of research is done into longevity. We try everything to live longer and we are becoming good at it. I heard somebody say once, on a conference about longevity, that the first person that will become a thousand years old has already been born. Almost all body parts are replaceable already and what we don't control yet we will probably learn and apply within the next 100 years. That is a scary thought. In order to preserve life, people have to die. What is going to happen if more and more people are getting older and older? Who is going to decide who will live another 100 years or will die right away? There are already 6 billion people in the world, fighting and killing each other. Do we really need more? So what about stem cell use and DNA manipulation? We all want our loved ones to live forever, but the problem is that everybody wants that. Would you like to live in a world with, lets say, 15 billion people? There will be no more individuality. So really, this cannot happen, but the researchers will not stop and experiments will continue. Eventually it will be life itself that interferes. There will be other diseases and catastrophes and people will die until balance will be restored. The earth will simply shake its skin, like a wet dog, and all that is not necessary will fall off.

Too many people and no individuality mean that in case of sickness the treatment will also not be individual. There is more and more specialisation and we cannot see the person behind the sickness anymore; **we can't see the patient for the trees.**

A good example comes to mind. A test was done with a patient with lower back pain. This patient was sent to 5 different specialists and ended up with 5 different diagnoses. The surgeon said that it was coming from the kidneys and wanted to operate, because that is what he does. The chiropractor said that it was a misalignment of the spine and wanted to make an adjustment, because that is what he does. The physiotherapist said it was a muscle spasm and wanted to give exercises, because that is what he does. The general practitioner said it was based on osteoarthritis of the vertebrae and prescribed medication, because that is what he does. And finally the psychologist said it was coming from stress and wanted to give a relaxation therapy, because that is what he does.

In the end the patient was confused and the complaints were still there and nobody had taken the time to look at this particular patient and his background and circumstances. Nobody had been able to make a diagnosis, based on the combined social, physical and emotional factors that made this patient who he was.

As a result wrong diagnoses are made and wrong treatments are started. Like a patient of mine with headache, ear ringing and blurry vision, since a few months. During intake he was telling about a lot of stress in his life, in his relationship and financial troubles. He was deeply worried. He visited an eye specialist who absolutely could not see the connection and only concentrated on the eyes.

Or a patient with neck pain, bad posture, limited mobility in the neck, repetitive activity in work, computer work, who develops arm- and wrist pain. His doctor referred him to a surgeon, who performed surgery for Carpal Tunnel Syndrome. His complaints got worse.

Another patient experienced pain in the Achilles tendon. In the assessment he spoke about long term back pain on the same side, plus numbness and tingling in the leg. The Achilles tendon looked great. The problem was sciatic pain. The medical diagnosis was Achilles tendonitis.

When I was working on cruise ships I had a standard questionnaire for intake of the patient. I always asked if patients were taking prescription medication and in 60% of the cases people were taking meds for high blood pressure, cholesterol, gastric reflux, diabetes type 2 and thyroid. It looked like it was standard procedure whether they were actually suffering from it or not.

It also means that the body itself is not going to do anything anymore, because it is getting whatever it needs. That is a very important thing to remember. Bodies, like all living things, have a tendency to become lazy. If it does not need to do something, it won't. If certain chemicals are necessary for normal functioning it will produce them. If for some reason the production stagnates or stops – stress for example – we can add these chemicals artificially, but by doing so we also suppress the body's own ability to produce it and the longer this situation lasts, the harder it is to fix. Think for example about high blood pressure: why would the body regulate that if it gets medication year after year? It says thank you very much and leans back and does nothing and eventually develops sickness, because of the unnecessary intake of toxic chemicals. Sooner or later that is going to happen.

We have to look at these things in perspective. Many patients need to take medication and that is the benefit of modern medicine, but at the same time billions of dollars worth of overprescribed drugs are wasted yearly and are affecting our health adversely.

Summary

We are living in a complex world with less norms and values. That leads to degeneration and people tend to isolate themselves and don't participate. The result can be sickness and addictions. Because we realize that we are doing something wrong we try to compensate, for example with visits to the gym and diet change, but we often go too fast. Our body will give warning signs, but it is hard to listen, especially because everybody does it and we want to be part of the group.
A good way to learn to listen is to use meditation.
Our medical system is so specialised that the individual patient is often overlooked. Too much medication is prescribed and our bodies get lazy and don't know how to heal anymore.

*The Results Of Any Medical Treatment
Are Proportional To How Well The Patient Is
Treated By The Practitioner*

Chapter 4

Medical Awareness

So, how difficult is it to be our own doctor? Above all, it is a matter of common sense. Our body is constantly giving feedback; that is the beauty of it: it will always react on what we put in it and what we do with it. It can be very subtle or very blunt, but we can always be aware of the reaction. If we are thirsty and we drink water, our thirst will be quenched, we are even minded and energized and we will have a regular bowel movement, just to name a few reactions. If we pay attention, we can notice all those effects and we feel balanced.

If we are thirsty and we drink pop, our thirst will initially be quenched, but soon we are thirsty again, we easily become hyper and over-energized, followed by tiredness, because of the refined sugar boost in our blood, our bowel movement will eventually stagnate, because the sugar overloads our digestive system and we will get constipation. Our metabolism will change and we will start gaining weight. All these effects are noticeable, if we pay attention.

We usually don't pay attention, because some of the effects don't show right away and because we become sugar addicts, pop addicts. It is amazing how many people are addicted to soft drinks. So we keep taking these refined sugars and keep poisoning our body. We know the consequences, but we don't listen.

An unhealthy lifestyle, with a bad diet, lack of movement, smoking, (over) use of alcohol, will eventually lead to cardiovascular problems, like heart attacks and strokes. Long before this actually happens there are all kinds of signs and warnings that the body is giving us, for example tiredness and lack of stamina, not sleeping well, weight gain, irritation, feelings of depression, digestive disorders etc. Many people say that a few days before they had a stroke, they felt a sudden numbness in one of their arms, or there was a short, acute, severe headache. These are ultimate signs and often it is already too late. We often don't recognise these symptoms for what they are, but they are definitely there and if we would listen and take action we would be able to prevent a lot of serious problems.

What makes it more challenging for us to be proactive is the fact that in the west we are not used to be preventive when it comes to health care, at least we weren't for the longest time. We always visit the doctor when something is already going on, when the symptoms start to interfere with our participation in the rat race. These symptoms are often the tip of the iceberg and it took years of misuse to get there. Now we get sick and we expect to get better soon and that the medication will take care of it. For some reason, we *are* preventive with the health of our teeth. We visit the dentist every 6 months, to prevent dental problems, but not in regular health care. The reason, I believe, that we are not proactive is because we totally trust in medication, the doctor and our whole healthcare system to make us better, when something is wrong. This is also what the system always has promoted. We were not supposed to know or understand anything about our own health, let alone do something about it. I was born in 1950 in the Netherlands and I remember well that my parents totally trusted everything about their or our health to the doctor. Doctors – general practitioners- in Europe were and still are used to do lots of home visits, especially in those days, so they often are well known and appreciated friends of the family and medical opinions, diagnoses and decisions are made in the warm, friendly atmosphere of the house and rarely questioned. In those years nobody was really concerned with their health, when it came to diet and physical activity. Gyms and sport schools were practically nonexistent and the very few people who did some kind of workout were often seen as weird. Everybody smoked everywhere; I remember going to the doctor and he received me in his office, sitting behind a big desk with a spilling ashtray in front of him and a burning cigarette between his fingers, while he asked me, deeply inhaling, what he could do for me. Many of my high school teachers were chain smokers in the classroom and even my dance instructor taught us the jive, while dancing with one of my classmates with a cigarette in his mouth.

My father died at the age of 52 from a stroke and of course we were all shocked, so young and unexpected. Later we realised that he had all the ingredients necessary to get a stroke: overweight, heavy smoker, no physical activity whatsoever, and probably high blood pressure. We just did not pay attention, because we thought it was normal.

It lasted until the nineteen seventies and eighties before working-out became widely accepted. Arnold Schwarzenegger was in top form during the seventies and helped developing bodybuilding and body awareness in general. Gyms and sport schools started to appear here and there and in the eighties and nineties people became more and more aware of the importance of a good diet. Since the start of the new millennium working-out, dieting and body awareness have not only become common good, but also soon turned into a social madness. So, from doing nothing, we went to becoming aware and eventually to doing too much.

We are living in a world, as I mentioned before, where individuality and personality are dominated by performance, money, power and social status and almost everybody is involved. It is standard and sucks us in, so that we can participate to get appreciation and respect. It is a world where both our physical- and mental health are subject to social success. This is an unnatural situation, because at the end of the day we are first and foremost individuals, who like to live in balance with our self and with nature that surrounds us. Therefore a national feeling of guilt is developing, because we need that balance, but at the same time we know that we will never be able to find it running along with the rest. So, to satisfy this feeling of guilt we are looking for ways to find "balance". One of the things we think are very important is to work on our body: we start working-out, drinking water and changing our diet. Of course, all of these things are good, when you look at it separately, but our feeling of guilt is so strong that we start overdoing it.

Gyms and sport schools are everywhere; every self-respecting family has at least two memberships, because to admit to friends and coworkers that we are not working-out is social suicide. I ask most of my patients if they are doing a sport or if they work out, just because I want to know if they are, because that might have an effect on the treatment. People always apologize if they are not, and they shouldn't. Many times these people are more in balance than a lot of gym members.

Working-out creates endorphins and makes us feel good. And we can definitely become addicted to our own endorphins. The more endorphins the better, people seem to think, but there can also be too much of it. Why would a person, let's say, 30 years old, a job, a family, a mortgage, car payments, worries etc. decide to run a marathon, 42 plus kilometers? That seems crazy, 4 hours at least of sweating, heart racing, exhaustion, cramping and mental challenge for what? We only do that, because of the endorphins, we love the endorphins, they drug us and keep us going, without endorphins marathons would be an affair of a couple of diehards. Is running a marathon balancing, when we are not a member of the Masai and when we don't need to hunt for our food for our survival? Maybe, when we always have done it and we have lots of time to relax and to recover, when our diet is in balance with our natural surroundings, instead of taking energy foods and vitamin waters, maybe then it is balancing, but not for the majority of marathon runners. I love to run, have been doing it since I was 25, but now, at 63, I run two to three times per week 5 km with my dog, more jogging than running. I feel good with it and I feel balanced. I am not tired or having muscle reactions and it feels like I can keep doing it forever. In my clinic I often treat people my age who run marathons or half marathons and they always develop complaints, because they don't listen to the signs and signals of their body. Our body will always let us know if we are doing the right thing. Of course, this worldwide problem of over-exercising has everything to do with stress as a logical consequence of the constant urge to perform and score. Stress, although nowadays seen as a bad thing, is in itself just a natural reaction of the body on something threatening. As the caveman wants to run away from the cave bear that threatens his existence, we want to run away from the social demands and expectations. In both cases, the body switches into survival mode, meaning that our vital organs, like heart, brain and muscles, need extra oxygen. Our endocrine system releases several chemicals like adrenaline and cortisol to do this. When used to escape the threatening situation, everything will calm down and we are fine, but in the modern world we have continuous situations that threaten our balance, it never stops. So, the production of these hormones continues as well and because we don't use everything, they remain in our body and eventually become toxic. That leads to a multitude of symptoms, like inflammation, depression, tiredness, sleep disturbances, mood swings, and... too much exercise. That's right, too much exercise is a symptom of stress, of a body that is not in balance. Because we want that balance, one way or another, we try to reach it by producing more endorphins. In other words, we try to cure an unnatural situation with an addiction, in fact exactly the same thing a drug addict does. The only cure is, of course, not to get into that unnatural situation in the first place.

Although there are lots of negative side effects from overtraining, it at least comes from a desire to live a healthier lifestyle and when we learn how to channel it properly it can only lead to something good. This is not the case when we look at recent changes in the health care system itself, which is showing all kinds of signs that it wants to do more about prevention. That itself is a good thing of course, but to achieve it by over testing and over screening and the prescription of medication or performing of surgery based on the outcome is again too mechanical and not directed to the person of the patient. It has nothing to do with living a healthier lifestyle, because, again, it leaves our wellbeing in the hands of machines and medication. Apart from an occasional course of antibiotics, I have never taken any prescription medication for a prolonged period of time. I also know that the majority of my childhood friends (baby boomers) have never done so. We all grew up in Europe and they must have another take on medication over there. After our immigration to Canada I noticed an increased use of medication among the people there, but when I worked as an acupuncturist on cruise ships for three years, where the majority of the guests were from the USA, I was shocked about the amount of prescription medication Americans are taking and then mainly, as I mentioned before, for high blood pressure, cholesterol levels (statins), acid reflux, diabetes type 2 and thyroid. At some point I could almost predict, when a 50 or 60-year-old American male came in, what medication he was using. For me, this was another proof of how the system does not look at the person, but at the disease, and in these cases not even at the disease, but at the possibility that it might develop in the future. Most of all it seemed to come from over-advertising of medication and scaring people into believing that without taking them they would almost certainly get sick. Flu shots are a good example of this principle. For years we all lived without flu shots and occasionally got sick and of course occasionally some older people or young children would become a victim of a flu infection. But that still does not justify the craze about flu shots these days. The pushy advertising campaigns and worldwide scaring of people to take it or face the consequences are so clearly orchestrated by the pharmaceutical industry that you have to be blind to miss it. I remember working for a hospital as a physiotherapist and when flu season arrived a nurse came by all departments with a cart full of flu syringes. When I refused I almost lost my job.

Being aware of the unhealthy lifestyle we are living, many of us feel guilt and start eating salads and over-exercising and others, who don't really want to change their lifestyle, feel the need to do something and start taking preventive medication; by doing so they expose themselves to an endless list of side effects, without stimulating their body to self regulation. For example, side effects for most cholesterol level regulating drugs are:

- muscle pain and damage,
- liver damage,
- digestive problems like nausea, gas, diarrhoea, constipation,
- skin rash,
- flushing,
- increased blood sugar or type 2 diabetes and
- neurological signs like memory loss and confusion.

Those for high blood pressure are:
- drowsiness,
- kidney area and lower back pain,
- dry cough,
- dizziness,
- faintness,
- light-headedness,
- skin rash.

For acid reflux (PPI's):
- bone fractures,
- bacterial infections,
- reduction of absorption of nutrients,
- pneumonia.

For diabetes type 2:
- stomach upset,
- skin rash,
- weight gain,
- kidney problems,
- tiredness,
- dizziness,
- gas and diarrhoea,
- anaemia,
- swelling ankles and
- low blood sugar.

For thyroid:
- abdominal cramps,
- diarrhoea,
- headache,
- heat intolerance,
- sleep disturbances,
- sweating,
- weight loss and
- diabetes type 2.
-

So many regularly prescribed drugs to prevent certain diseases have other diseases as side effects. Symptoms are suppressed, but not annihilated and a lifetime of medication use is waiting. This is exactly what the pharmaceutical industry wants, because they are more interested in selling products than healing a disease. Diabetes, high blood pressure, GERD and high cholesterol are all examples of big, multibillion-dollar businesses, and we, the people, let it all happen.

British Columbia, Canada, established in 1994 the Therapeutics Initiative, an organisation run out of the University of British Columbia in Vancouver to check efficiency and safety of prescription drugs. This organisation has been a thorn in the eyes of pharmaceutical companies and since a year its funding has been reduced by the government and access to necessary patient data has become more and more difficult. In other words, one of the few independent organisations that can give us unbiased information about what we should be swallowing is slowly being strangled, because it interferes with the profits of the big pharmaceutical money-makers.

Why are we accepting all this? Why are we so meek and inactive when it comes to our health? Why are we so alert and sharp when we need to spend money on consumer goods, read all kinds of tests about a vehicle we want to buy, negotiate with the salesman about better price and warranty? Why do we accept everything the doctor says, even if it has great impact on our personal, daily and financial life? Ignorance and fear for our wellbeing are main factors, but aren't we ignorant as well about cars, electronics, computers, washers and dryers, just to name a few?

If a product causes us any discomfort or damage we bring it back to the manufacturer and demand replacement or a refund and most companies hurry to comply in fear of creating a bad reputation and because they want to stand behind their products, yet if a medication causes us severe headaches, nausea and muscle ache, interfering with our daily lives, our relationships and ability to work, we just accept it. It does not make sense at all and it is time we change and become critical consumers of everything others want us to buy in the health care field. It is time to use the information sources that are so readily available to anyone on the Internet.

Health care, hospitals, clinics, MRI's, X-rays, blood tests and so on are all just part of a business model, and we can decide to buy or not, just as we can buy consumer goods and services, or not. As a postwar child from Europe it took me also a while to get used to that idea, but that is basically all it is. Because health care affects us all, parts of it are funded and subsidized, but it is still a business model. The manager of a hospital used to be a doctor, now it is somebody with a business degree. A surgeon rents space and equipment from a hospital, so he wants to do enough surgeries to be able to pay his bills and make some profit. More and more private clinics, MRI stations and labs are emerging and they all want to make money.

There is so much information out there about every drug we can think of, every medical procedure we might become subjected to, every existing disease or medical condition, that we are able to form a well-founded opinion and ask clear questions. There are websites where we can type in the name of any drug and read about its effects, side effects, alternatives and safety (for example RxISK.org). After we have informed our self we can make an appointment with our doctor and know exactly what to ask and what to suggest. Many insurance companies offer the option to go for a second opinion. If we go to a restaurant and we don't like the food, the service or the staff, we don't go there anymore. If we go to see a specialist about our health it is important to understand and like each other, because it is about our health, the greatest good we possess. If we don't like the person, the way of handling and the feedback, we should go somewhere else. Maybe we'll have to travel a bit further, but it might be worth it. Don't get overwhelmed or impressed by the doctor, because it is our body, our money and our future. We can see that the attitude is already changing, because they have to; we, the patients, are starting to not accept it anymore. Don't forget that health care professionals can do their jobs, because of us, are earning an income, because of us. Without us, there would be no health care practitioners.

Ask to explain everything in clear language and don't accept vague talk or technical jargon with colleagues about our condition in our presence.

Things to ask are:

- What exactly is my problem?
- What is the prognosis?
- What can I do myself to make it better?
- What is the medication doing?
- What are the side effects of the medication?
- How long do I need to take this medication?
- Is surgery really the only solution?

- What are the consequences of surgery?
- Will I fully recover or will there be permanent changes in my condition?

It is time to re-educate the health care practitioners, especially medical specialists. Medical specialists are the end station in their medical field and nobody can correct them or control them, at least not in matters concerning their specialisation. So it is our opinion and gut feeling against their expertise, and both sides should acknowledge that, not just us. A good healthcare practitioner listens very well and pays a lot of attention to our opinion and gut feeling. If he doesn't and just pushes through, based on the arrogance of his status and knowledge, he'll bring us out of balance and that would greatly affect the results of the treatment. I have learned that the hard way and now I really listen well and if I notice any kind of resentment or apprehension I talk it over or try to find an alternative, preferably an alternative, because normally apprehension does not go away after a conversation. When the patient is at ease, trusting and understanding what is going on, already 50% improvement is won. Apprehension and mistrust lead to a higher level of sympathetic activity in the autonomous nerve system and that means production of chemicals that make us stressed and then everything gets worse. I see these things happening almost every day. Because acupuncture is not yet fully integrated in mainstream medical care it needs to be introduced with tact and patience. People can be apprehensive at first and if I don't explain it right and don't take time to calm the patient down, he will get a negative experience and that forms his future look at it. It is very hard to erase a first negative experience, if you get a chance at all. So, I always explain and ask for consent and interpret the look in his eyes and the way he speaks. Doing it this way will almost always lead to a positive experience.

I am convinced that the results of any medical treatment are proportional to the way the patient is treated by the practitioner, whether trust and understanding are established and if respect towards the patient is shown. This goes for everything, whether it is an acupuncture treatment, that requires rest and relaxation or a highly technical surgical procedure, where the patient is out and not aware of the proceedings. Even if the procedure itself is technical, unattached and impersonal, proper preparation of the patient and reassurance are still important contributors to the end result. We are living beings with feelings and needs. All we want is to feel good. Whoever or whatever makes us feel good has already won. This is a very well known principle in many facets of life, especially in retail sales. If the client is happy, business will thrive. Nice offices, smiling salesmen, coffee, personal attention, a toy for the kids and going the extra mile, are all examples of making the client feel good. Businesses are spending a lot of money on courses and seminars to teach their staff how to sell and make the client happy. In fact, if we don't receive this kind of attention, we go somewhere else. Why is this not the same in the world of health and medical care? One of the most general surgeries, appendix removal, costs on average about $ 30,000.00 in the US. That is the price of a nicely equipped SUV. If we go to the dealer to order one we will be pampered and praised, if we go to the hospital we are number 37, are pushed out of the bed as soon as possible and are supposed to follow a protocol and nobody really cares about us. We are too humble and let it happen, and by doing that we reinforce the behaviour of healthcare practitioners and nothing will ever change.

I treated this lady with sleeping problems. She was suffering from insomnia for years already and taking daily sleeping pills. I treated her initially for a broken leg with acupuncture, a local treatment, but she already reacted positively with her whole body. When I heard about the sleeping problems I suggested treating her for that as well. After about 5 treatments with acupuncture she calmed down considerably, was sleeping a lot better and managed to reduce her sleeping medication with 50%. Before we started acupuncture, she visited a sleeping clinic in the hospital. She was tested and one of the outcomes was that her brain showed too much activity during sleep (why?); she was aroused as they put it. They suggested starting some exercises and after 6 weeks she was supposed to go down with her medication. When she told the practitioner that she was receiving acupuncture since a few weeks and already went 50% down with her medication and was doing well, the answer was that that was not the protocol they used and that she was to proceed with what they advised.

The protocol was more important than the patient. The proper reaction would have been to be happy for her and tell her that she should continue her acupuncture treatments and that she could come back if in the end it would not help her enough.

I understand that the huge supply of patients who visit a hospital requires rules and regulations, but eventually it is about the well being of these patients, however that is achieved. All those people with complaints, who never enter an acupuncture clinic, obviously have chosen to go into the mainstream care system and that is fine. They obviously feel at ease and comfortable with that way of treatment and that is what it is all about. I understand that, as a non-mainstream practitioner, and I will encourage it, but what about the other way around? When will a surgeon say, why don't you first try to do some acupuncture before I put my knife in you? Or the GP, why don't you go for yoga and relaxation and become physically active, before I prescribe these antidepressants?

The main reasons are ignorance about what other disciplines can do, arrogance, fear of competition, abuse of power and the general notion among the public that the doctor knows best. There is no cooperation for the benefit of the patient. The patient should be in the centre and there should be mutual referrals, but unfortunately the system, the protocols and the money are central and the patient is the victim.

Most research money goes into mainstream care; there is not a lot of money available for research into the effects of acupuncture, meditation, diet change and relaxation, to name a few. We are living in a time of numbers, proof, evidence and testing and only then something is right. Whether or not the patient reacts well is not the issue, there should be evidence. If there is evidence, maybe there will be some money.

What I am trying to say is, that if we treat a human being in a way a human being deserves, he will react well, start to heal and find balance again. We don't need evidence, testing and numbers to see that somebody is doing well. Some insurers require range of motion measurement numbers for the different joints that are being treated. So if the shoulder moves to 90 degrees now and started at 70 degrees, the patient is doing better and it is worth paying for. Whether or not the patient feels better is less important. I cannot count the cases anymore where the patient's wellbeing was not proportional with the range of motion of his injured joint.

It would be very interesting to see a large, government funded, properly set up study into the overall effects of de-stressing and relaxation on any kind of disease or health condition. The outcome could reduce the general healthcare expenses considerably.

There are other medical systems in the world that *are* very preventive, like Oriental medicine. Many people in China and other Asian countries visit an acupuncturist on a regular basis, just for what I call a tune-up treatment. Tune-up treatments are not about treating certain health conditions, but are meant to keep the body healthy and in balance. A limited amount of the strongest working acupuncture points is used to boost the immune system and to balance the autonomic nervous system.

These treatments can be found everywhere; they are simple, fast, cheap and effective. If these treatments, about twice per year, are combined with a conscious lifestyle, a good diet and regular physical activity they can greatly reduce the services of modern medicine and generate huge savings in health care. They also are part of the recipe to become 100 years old in good health.

This can only be done, when people are willing to change their way of life. Oriental people usually have a stronger sense of holistic living than we here in the West. In modern China traditional medicine has an official place in health care next to modern medicine and people can choose between the two. Many still rely on the benefits and experience of traditional medicine.

What it all comes down to is a lack of balance. Balance is not an integral part of our western lifestyle. It is therefore more difficult for us to implement it in our lives.

Summary

We should pay attention to the feedback our body is giving us and be proactive, but because we trust our medical system to fix us when something goes wrong, proactivity is not our strongest point. Other health care systems can be more preventive, like Chinese medicine.

Awareness about health is growing and we start to live more consciously, but we have the tendency to overdo it, either with too much exercise or with the use of preventive medication, with all its side effects.

We should start looking at ourselves as customers instead of patients and be just as critical towards the products the health industry is trying to sell us as we are towards consumer goods.

Lots of information about health and sickness is readily available on the Internet and we should use that to our advantage.

We should try to introduce more balance into all aspects of our lives. It would make us so much healthier.

We Need To Interact With Each Other
In Order To Establish
A Mutually Beneficial Relationship

Chapter 5

Reasons to be our own doctor

Being our own doctor has so many advantages. Before we are going to look at them there are a few points of order. As I said in the beginning, this is not a crusade against modern medicine. Modern medicine can be a lifesaver and is very good in the treatment of acute conditions. It also has the ability to look inside the body and make physical changes that otherwise are not possible. Any medical condition can always end up in such a situation and then we should use what modern medicine has to offer. But before we dive into the system, we want to be sure that we did everything to stimulate our own body to heal. We want to be sure that we understand as much as possible about our medical condition, so that we can make responsible decisions and leave to the professional what we cannot treat our self. That is the purpose of this book, to make us aware of what makes us sick, how we can recognize it and how we can stimulate our body and mind to fix it.

1. *Responsibility – A Good Thing*

For me, as a baby boomer, the lack of responsibility these days is mind-boggling. I was raised with so much emphasis on the fact that we were responsible for our actions, that it became a second nature. Having responsibility is not something we have to like per se, and it is always a nice feeling, if something bad happens, to know that we are not responsible. It also has positive qualities, because if something good happens, it is a nice feeling to know that we are responsible for all that goodness. It gives us respect, appreciation and admiration and we all crave that. In the superficial world we live in these days, we try everything to not be responsible, especially here in North America. In Europe, at least until recently, we could get away with a lot of things that would be a reason for suing here. Punitive damages did not really exist and most situations would be described in a law book and carry a maximum amount of money. The result was that people there accepted that 'shit happens' and went on with their lives. Here a simple mistake can sometimes ruin somebody's life.

Reluctantly, we accept responsibility in those cases, where there is no way around it, but being responsible for our own health is still something we not readily accept. Most of the time we feel it is not our fault when we get sick or fall or get involved in an accident, and it certainly is not our responsibility to heal from it. That is usually left in the hands of health care practitioners. That is the way it was taught. That is also what we can find in the old Hippocratic oath, the ancient adagium doctors still live by: 'I will prescribe regimens for the good of my patients according to my ability and my judgment...'

The doctor will prescribe and the patient undergoes. I remember this old lady in the Netherlands, living alone in a little apartment. I was asked to make a house call. In older Dutch houses, you ring the bell, the door opens and when you step in there is immediately a flight of stairs and the inhabitant usually stands at the top of the stairs to see who is coming in. After I announced myself and started to climb up the stairs she told me that she had already seen 14 different practitioners for her complaints and that she did not have much confidence in my abilities. The first thing that went through my mind was, ok, so I am number 15; that is all I am. She was defiant and put the load of her problems on my shoulders before I even got in, and made my trip upstairs even harder. I was a lot younger in those days and initially I accepted that she was pointing to me as the one who had to solve her problem. That did not work of course and after a few treatments I told her that it was not my problem, but hers and if she would not accept that, her complaints would never get better. I even told her that the fact that she was still suffering so much from this condition was because she never took possession of it. The next thing I know was that she abstained from any more treatments. It was a woman alone, lacking social contact, using the medical system to get attention and continuing the process with every next helper until someone finally put a stop to it. Of course, she felt attacked. It never entered her mind, that she was responsible.

Of course, being involved in a fall or motor vehicle accident does not happen by choice, but the consequences of it are our responsibility. I have felt many times that people came by and acted like: "here is my arm; it hurts there. I will come by on my way back and pick it up".

Our health is our responsibility. The health care practitioner will explain and guide us through the process, but it is our problem.

2. Satisfaction

Usually when we leave things in the hands of somebody else it doesn't help us build up our self-esteem. Going to a doctor and waiting for a diagnosis is a passive thing that does not involve our own decision making. We just have to believe that what he is saying is true. If we can find out what is wrong with us, by noticing symptoms, looking it up online and eliminating other options, we feel satisfied. It is a good feeling, knowing that we can do that and if a visit to the doctor is necessary, we come prepared and can ask the right questions.

I went to a doctor once with an infection on one of my fingers. It had been infected for a long time and did not want to get any better. I had hoped that the doctor would open it up by piercing it, so that the pus would come out. In stead, he gave me a prescription for antibiotics and obviously did not feel like touching it. I ignored the prescription and went home. I sat under a lamp and had a good look at my finger with a magnifying glass. I took a heated needle and pushed it through the skin and a minute later pus came out and the problem was fixed. I had saved myself from taking drugs and fixed the problem in a blink. That was very satisfying.

3. Confidence

Just as being able to figure out something our self is very satisfying, it also helps building our confidence. If we did it once we might be able to do it again. Confidence supports our feeling of self-respect. People like to be among people who show confidence. It gives them a feeling of safety, a feeling that when something goes wrong they will fix it. Confident people also carry that feeling over on others. They make other people also more confident.

Our health is pretty important and to be able to have a guiding hand in it is certainly strengthening our confidence.

4. Independence

Independence is one of the greatest values in life. Not having to wait for somebody else and not having to hope that the other person is doing the right thing, in fact not having to doubt if the other person has the proper knowledge, is a relief and gives a feeling of freedom. Especially when it comes down to our health. Our health is our greatest good and other people can so easily talk about it and dismiss our concerns. We don't have to wait for the doctor's office to be open; we don't have to wait in crowded waiting rooms. We can just sit down and browse the Internet, talk to friends or relatives and determine if what we have is a valid reason to visit the doctor. It is surprising how much we can find online and how much it can reassure us that it is nothing serious. Don't forget: about 80% of the issues we can develop are being taken care of by our body and don't need a doctor's attention. The British Medical Journal stated in 2012 that in the US alone unnecessary medical care totaled up to 800 billion dollars per year.
It is also important to stay away from repetitive treatments by different healthcare providers. If we go to a physiotherapist, chiropractor, acupuncturist or massage therapist, we should insist on a treatment plan and a time frame. In general we can say that an evaluation should be made after 5 to 6 treatments. If no change in the condition is visible it is probably not going to work and we either have to stop or do a reassessment. Never concede to a permanent maintenance program, because it makes the body lazy, depending on the passive input by the practitioner and it will not stimulate the body to heal. I know some chiropractors that believe that people have to come in for life to get adjustments done on their spine to prevent them from developing problems, even young children. That cannot be right. A therapist or doctor is there

to guide the patient through the process of getting and staying better and above all, to involve the patient in his own health, not to make them depending on their treatments. That is usually better for their own wallets than for their patient's wellbeing.

5. Self-respect – The Manna Of Life

Being respectful to our self, means that we value us for what we are worth and that we are proud of the things we have accomplished in our life. It does not matter at what level. It is absolutely unimportant whether we became famous or rich or the CEO of a big company. It is all about the fact that we have actually done something with our life. I know too many people who don't have that feeling of self-respect. They always find whatever they have done mediocre and assume that others feel the same. It is like minimalizing a screen on a computer: click on the minus and we disappear into the lower right corner, where we live a modest life in the background. I don't mean to say that we should be the opposite, loud, boasting and always too present. Those people are horrible, they don't listen to what anybody has to say and only want to showcase themselves. We should find a position in centre, where we are seen, but not ostentatiously.
Self-respect is the engine that keeps us going. It stimulates us to make the best of our selves and it keeps challenging us to go on.
If we have lived a life full of self-respect, then, at the end of the day, we can look back and be satisfied.
Being our own doctor is very satisfying and makes us appreciate ourselves more. Another very important consequence of being self-respective is that we automatically respect others more for what they have

accomplished. It builds a better world.

6. *Becoming Aware Of Our Body*

We can only notice something that might be going on in our body if we listen to it. Listening to their body is for many people a new thing and difficult in the beginning. Many people also don't have a strongly developed body 'feel'. All kinds of things can be going on in our body and we might have no idea. Most of us, who are not involved in any medical profession or sport, have never learned how to be aware of body signs.

Let us just take a simple example. Posture, good posture, is a very important thing, because bad posture can lead to many nasty complaints. Certain degenerative changes are taking place in the body anyway, but will become worse and develop faster if we have bad posture. For example osteoarthritis, a thinning of the cartilage of the bones that already starts in our thirties, becomes worse when we are over 50. It has a preference to go to the neck, lower back, hips, knees and finger joints. The discs between the vertebrae of the spine become thinner, there is more pressure on the little connecting joints and nerve compression can be the result. When we sit and work on a computer a lot or when we are driving long distances on a regular basis our posture becomes bad: our head slides forward, putting even more pressure on the joints and the shoulder joints also move forward, limiting their range of motion and increasing the chance of inflammation. So, bad posture speeds up the osteoarthritis process. But many people don't even know that they have bad posture.

We need to learn to recognize the signs that our body is giving us. Neck pain because of osteoarthritis starts as a stiffness and limited range of motion and is usually worse in the morning. It can also lead to numbness and tingling in the arms and hands. If we feel something like that and we are also aware that our working posture is bad, we know almost for certain what the cause is. We also know then that going to the doctor would be unnecessary, because the solution is changing our posture and becoming more active. The doctor would probably prescribe medication for the pain and order an X-ray. Medication would probably not be necessary if we change our habits and an X-ray would only confirm what we already know, namely osteoarthritis of the neck. We have saved our self a visit to the doctor, saved the medical system an unnecessary X-ray and money for medication.

This is just one simple example of something that might be going on in our body and that can be fixed by awareness and willingness to make changes.

Another thing that comes from body awareness is the possibility of feeling the level of seriousness of the situation. We all know what an oncoming cold feels like, like having a sore throat, coughing, maybe a light fever and phlegm formation. We recognize that and at the same time know that it is not serious, if we take the proper precaution measures. In fact most of us don't even think about visiting the doctor when we feel a cold starting. The reason is that we recognize it and don't have to worry.

If the cold would be untreated or neglected it could turn into pneumonia (lung infection). Common signs of pneumonia are deep cough, fever, chills, chest pain, fast heartbeat, tiredness and a general weak feeling. When we experience that, we know that it is more serious and a visit to the doctor is necessary.

The more we are focused on what is happening inside our body, the more we recognize so that we can take the necessary steps.

Body awareness is a valuable asset in trying to be our own doctor. It can be learned and practiced, just by staying alert.

7. Stimulate Our Body To Heal

By recognizing what is going on in our body and by taking the necessary steps to improve the situation, we stimulate our body to heal. Once we have experienced an unpleasant situation with certain signs and symptoms, it leaves a footprint in our mind and the next time we know what is happening. Just like we can stimulate our body to recognize sickness, we can also stimulate it to heal. The self-healing capacity of the body is working all the time anyway. If we cut our finger the body will fix it, whether we want it or not. If we catch a cold our immune system will be activated and we get better in a few days. We can speed up this process by eating well, by taking enough rest, by meditating and concentrating on the affected part of our body. If we strongly believe that our body can take care of the problem it will usually happen. Why does an aspirin help against headache? Is that because the ingredients suppress pain, or improve blood circulation or relax the muscles? Or is it because we are so used to the fact that it takes care of our headache that we simply cannot imagine that it will not work? Isn't that the way the placebo effect works? I believe that, if I really would not believe that a Tylenol could help me, it will not help me. In other words, drugs cause certain chemical reactions in our body, including the ones that are the result of our believing in their positive effect, and therefore they 'help'. But without our believe drugs would have a hard time. It is simply amazing how strong the influence of our minds can be, or of somebody else's mind, for that matter. It is a well-known fact that a caring and warm person, doctor or not, can have a very healing effect on our health.

Let me give you an example. When I studied Traditional Chinese Medicine in the Netherlands, more than 30 years ago, equal minded doctors or other patients referred people to our clinic. First, a Western educated physician, who did an assessment, took pulse and blood pressure and spent about 30 minutes with them. During that time the patient had the chance to talk about his problem and, because it was an educational institution, he had all the attention. After the first encounter with the doctor, the patient was sent to us, the acupuncturists-hopeful. We did another assessment, elaborately, and gave the patient another hour of our time, asking questions and, above all, listening. Then the treatment started, checked many times by the supervisors and us. In the end the patient had had about two hours of undivided attention and was able to tell his story over and over again. Almost always that procedure healed about 60% of the problem.

We crave attention. A lot of our problems exist because we don't get the attention we deserve. I cannot remember how many times patients of mine have been waiting for months for an appointment with a specialist, expecting solutions and a listening ear, but coming out of the treatment room 5 minutes later, frustrated and disappointed. They did not get the attention they deserved.

Who can better give attention to our problems than us? We will always be our best doctors ever, because we understand our problems best.

8. Bring Balance In Our Body

Balance is the conditio-sine-qua-non of life. Without balance nothing works. It is already such an old adagium, but for some reason we seem to have forgotten about balance in modern life. Nature is the prime example of balance. Think about day and night, warm and cold, summer and winter, spring and fall, man and woman and so on. So the ingredients to live a balanced life are there; now we need to do something with it. The Western economic model of supply and demand shows a balanced starting point, but the people who need to execute it show no balance. There is too much stress, too much pressure, too many expectations, and too much emphasis on money and no pity or empathy. The things we do to balance this chaos are weak at best. We try to forcefully relax in the weekend and cram too many activities in too little time. We run and exercise, go to parties, drink too much and laugh too hard. All this is meant to be relaxing, but in reality it is still a form of hyper activity.

What we really need after a week of stress is quiet and silence, meditation, light and nutritious food, yoga exercises, sleeping, a good conversation with family or friends. That would bring some balance back.

We also have a typical Western approach to balance. Take our diet for example. Lets divide foods for the sake of balance in hot and cold. Meat, fish, eggs and alcohol are on the hot side, then we get fruits, vegetables and grains in the center and sweets, sugar and water are on the cold side. We tend to eat a lot of meat, fish and eggs. We like to swallow that away with alcohol. Our portions of vegetables and grains are usually small. We finish our meal with sweets, like deserts.

So if we put the food on a teeter-totter, then the hot food will be on one side and the cold food on the other. Now we think that we had a balanced meal. But the real balance of a teeter-totter is not at the ends but in the center, where the fruits, vegetables and grains are.

This is our idea of balance. Fix the stress with a workout in the gym or a highly competitive game of golf.

We simply don't know anymore what balance is and therefore we get sick, because our body and mind are still looking for that balance.

Oriental people always have had a much stronger sense of balance than we. They are much more connected with nature around them. I call that magic. They still see the magic. At least I hope that they will still be able to see that for a long time, because what is currently happening in China and India is not very encouraging.

Magic is all around us. We can see it in the trees and the flowers, we can hear it in the wind, smell in the air and touch it in the water of a river or an ocean. Magic is also present in us and if we let it, it can be a very powerful presence.

Most oriental ways of healing are based on balance. In acupuncture it is all about yin and yang. Everything in life is divided between yin and yang. Yin is the calm and passive factor and stands for cold and quiet, rest and relaxation, contemplation, meditation and sleep. Yang is the opposite; it is the hot and active factor and stands for heat and fire, anger and tension, frustration and impatience and for stress and restlessness. One cannot exist without the other; there is no day without a night, no man without a woman, no up without down and no water without fire. Looking at our daily way of life it is no surprise that we are a very yang society. It is therefore also no surprise that our diseases and medical conditions are also yang in character.

What the Chinese called yin and yang thousands of years ago, was based on their perception of the magic that surrounded them. They had no knowledge of the internal human body or the way the organs worked. Still their perception and interpretation was very close to the truth. We have two nervous systems in our body. We have the motoric nervous system that takes care of our movements. That is a voluntary system: we can decide to move or not, it is up to us. We also have the autonomic nervous system that takes care of everything else in our body. All the things that are out of our control, like blood pressure, blood circulation, functions of the organs, sleep regulation, temperature regulation and so on. This system is divided in an activating part and a deactivating part. The activating part is called the sympathetic system and the deactivating part is called the parasympathetic system. When we get scared our blood pressure goes up, our breathing becomes shallower and our heart rate goes up. We prepare for a fight or a flight. Our sympathetic system is dominating.

This is what the Chinese call yang. At night when we go to bed, the parasympathetic system takes over so that our blood pressure and heart rate can go down and we can breath easier; now the yin must dominate. These two systems have to be in balance. That is also what the body wants. Our body does not want to be out of balance, because it is an unnatural situation. It will try to get back in balance. That is also the self-healing property of our body. It is basically constantly trying to rebalance, no matter what we throw at it to do the opposite.

That self-healing, balancing capacity of our body is very strong, because it is part of our survival mechanism: if yin and yang are too far apart the body will die.

Looking at all the problems we get our self into, the constant struggle to stay balanced, we get an idea of how persistent we are in feeding our body and mind the wrong ingredients. I just read an article about the so-called Rushing Woman Syndrome. It points out that especially women overload themselves with work, chores and responsibilities, and therefore suffer a lot from depression and feelings of guilt. Whether or not it is a medical diagnose, it is a picture we can clearly recognize and we all know somebody in our circle of friends who fits in. We know we are out of balance and we know what to do about it and really don't need a doctor to confirm that. Balance is in our minds and we can feel it when it is there: mens sana in corpore sano, a healthy mind in a healthy body.

Luckily there are many different health care systems available these days, that are more balanced and more natural. Slowly people begin to understand and recognize these other ways of thinking, but it still has a long way to go. Traditional Chinese Medicine (TCM) is an example of a different approach.

When I started with my study in 1983 the use of acupuncture was still questionable, to say the least, and in some countries outright forbidden. People thought it was hocus-pocus and acupuncturists were generally seen as quacks. When I started to actually treat patients I used to spend at least an hour to explain, assess and treat. Because people were not familiar with the concept of Chinese medicine it was difficult to attract patients and therefore the price could not be too high. So, it was not really a lucrative business. Years later I met this Chinese practitioner here in Canada, who was highly successful with his treatments. It was refreshing to see how he promoted his profession and how he won people over. He set a very low price per treatment and sometimes even treated people for free the first time. He had all the confidence in the world and was genuinely convinced that he could help almost everybody. His goal was to make everybody feel better after the first treatment so that they would come back and he did everything he could to accomplish that. He was driven and invited everybody to come in. He gave people a feeling of confidence and reassurance and the waiting room was packed all the time. He never said no if somebody called. By creating this kind of atmosphere it was simply amazing how many people already felt better after the first time and how many really believed that they would get better by his treatments. That is how these things work. The body reacts on the input we give it. Read the Secret, if we really believe, it is going to happen. If we absolutely do not believe in the healing effect of a sleeping pill it is not going to help.

If somebody really does not believe in the effectiveness of acupuncture, stop pushing it, because it will not help this person.

The reason is that the use of whatever it is that we do not believe in, is not contributing to the internal balance that is needed to get better. In such a case surgery, for example, might, with all its negative side effects. We need to educate people to start believing in their own ability to heal and how to access that.

9. Be An Example And Stimulation For Others

Who does not know somebody who visits the doctor for everything? These are people who are very insecure and they need reassurance from the doctor that all is well. That will keep them going for a while and then it starts again. Whatever virus or bacteria is going around, they will get it and whatever illness or disease is being discussed on parties or in the media, they will develop the symptoms for sure.

We call them hypochondriacs. They always perceive the worst for themselves. People who had a stabile childhood with caring parents usually don't become hypochondriacs. But people who lacked attention will do everything to get it and going to the doctor is one way of doing it. It has a lot to do with the way we perceive the world around us.

By monitoring our self and recognizing signs and symptoms we become more secure and confident and maybe start worrying a little less.

Everybody can listen to their body and learn how to translate and interpret certain signals. The more apt we become in owning our body, the more we can stimulate others to do the same. It is so much more rewarding to do something our self instead of waiting for the results of what others do, whether it is about our health or something else.

10. Less Toxins In Our Body

There are so many reasons to be the guardian of our own health, but one of the most important ones is the reduction of getting toxic material in our body.

What exactly are toxins? I can give you a long and windy resume, but in short, toxins are chemicals that don't belong in our body, either because they have been added from outside for several reasons, or because our body produces them for a reason that never materializes.

Examples of toxins are polluted air, food additives like food dyes and chemical flavorings, water additives like chlorine and ammonia, chemicals like pesticides, mercury and paint thinners, but also body produced chemicals like adrenaline, noradrenaline and cortisol, also called stress hormones.

Thinking about this and then about a normal day in our lives, we can imagine that these toxins are attacking our body on a constant basis. There is practically nowhere to go in our modern society to stay out of the claws of toxins. One way would be to become a Tibetan monk, sit on a mountaintop cross-legged, and stare at our belly button for the best part of the day and think of nothing, but even that would not be a guarantee for a toxin-free environment.

Of course our body has defense mechanisms against things that float around and have no business there. The liver is a big filter that collects debris and gets rid of it. The kidneys do the same thing. Our lungs can also dispel toxic material and so does our skin. We normally get rid of toxins by expelling them via the intestines, as urine, or sweat and phlegm. As long as we have to deal with a moderate amount of toxic material we can handle it, but unfortunately, in this hectic life, there is no moderate amount. All processed foods contain toxins and just about all we eat is processed. It is very difficult and expensive to get organic food and almost impossible to make organic food the food source for the masses. We do our laundry with chemicals and clean the house with chemicals; we breathe polluted air and are under a constant load of stress.

Stress is a reason for our body to become alert, because it thinks that it is under attack. So, our brain thinks that it should defend our body. It releases stress hormones like adrenaline and cortisol. These chemicals are the reason for higher blood pressure, increased heart rate, shallow breathing, sweating etc. We need all that to save our live, to run from danger and in the process we burn those stress hormones out of our system. Problem solved. Except that in modern life that is not going to happen. We produce the same amount of stress hormone on a daily basis, for example by just crossing the street a few times, or trying to find a parking spot. The stress hormone that is released is present in our system, but it does not serve a purpose. So it becomes unwanted and toxic. Toxic material is being sent to the liver and other organs. The liver is a filter and can do only so much, before it becomes clogged. Now the toxins that cannot be expelled from our body are just floating around. Fat cells have the tendency to attract toxins and soon they will become surrounded by them. Now these cells are hard to approach. If we go for a workout and our body wants to burn fat to provide energy for our muscles, it cannot reach the fat cells. That is the reason why we can try to be very active, but still have a hard time losing weight. Another source of toxins are drugs and medication. They contain a lot of chemicals that the body has a hard time with to break down. I already mentioned how many drugs people in general and North Americans in particular are taking. We are constantly making our bodies sick with the negative side effects of stress and toxins and then try to fix it with even more toxins, while not making any changes in our lifestyle.

By being our own doctor we can drastically reduce the intake of toxins, not just by preventing the consumption of prescription drugs, but also by recognizing the signs and symptoms of too many toxins in our body and by taking our measures on time.

11. Less Inflammation In Our Body

Inflammation is starting to become a major cause of sickness. Research shows more and more conditions that started with inflammation: cardiovascular problems often start with an inflammation in the blood vessels, neurological conditions like MS and strokes are believed to have started as an inflammation in brain tissue. Many digestive disorders are based on inflammation. Inflammation is what the Chinese call a yang condition. There is too much heat in he body. Let us look at some very common health conditions and try to find out their character, whether they are hot or cold, yang or yin:

- *Headache*. Most headaches are bursting, giving a sensation of fullness in the head, get worse with stress (yang) and better with rest (yin). Headaches tend to get worse if the pressure increases, like bending over. Pressure is yang. In general the character of headache is yang or hot.
- ***GERD* or gastric reflux**. Patients are complaining about a burning feeling in the upper part of the stomach. Getting worse when eating greasy or spicy foods and when bending over. Sometimes they feel like vomiting. In Chinese medicine it is believed that the downward flow of the stomach energy is turning around and going up. All these are signs of heat. So the character of GERD is yang or hot.
- *Irritable Bowel Syndrome or IBS*. The bowels are irritated. Main symptoms are diarrhoea or constipation, bloating and gas, pain in the abdomen. Irritation in itself is already a sign of heat and bloating and gas are signs of high pressure. This is also a heat pattern. The general character of IBS is yang or hot.
- *Insomnia or sleeplessness*. At night our parasympathetic nerve system (yin) should prevail so that we can sleep. But if there is too much heat in the body it dominates and makes us stay awake at night. The character of insomnia is yang or hot.
- *High blood pressure*. The name explains itself. It gets worse under stress (yang) and when not taking enough rest (yin). The character of high blood pressure is yang or hot.
- *Tiredness*. Everybody is tired these days. It has the same explanation as insomnia and is a result of insomnia. Living a calm and balanced life doesn't tire us. The character of tiredness is yin, based on a reaction on too much yang.

- *Depression*. So many people suffer from depression. Depression is the result of a stressed and overloaded life, all signs of yang and heat. The character of depression is yin, based on a reaction on an overdose of yang.
- *Asthma*. Narrowing of the airways. Worse with stress (yang) and better with rest (yin). Asthma increases the pressure in the lungs. The character of asthma is yang or hot.
- *Allergies*. Symptoms are sneezing, watery and burning eyes, redness of the skin. All signs of heat. Allergies start when there are too many toxins in the body and toxins are yang in character. The character of allergies is yang or hot.

I can go on and on. In fact it is very difficult to come up with a disease that is yin in character. An example might be getting a severe cold, because of living in cold and wet circumstances and at the same time being very inactive. In the beginning this would be a condition of cold, but left untreated it would develop into something more serious, like pneumonia, and that is again yang in character. Inflammation is a situation in our body where our body tries to initiate a healing process by removing sick making factors, like bacteria or toxins. The classical signs of inflammation are rubor (redness), calor (heat), dolor (pain), tumor (swelling) and functio laesa (decreased function); all of them are signs of heat. Inflammation can go everywhere and researchers have found out that many more health issues are based on inflammation than we suspected. This is not a surprise, if we think about our daily life, filled with stressors and processed food and not taking enough rest and time for our self to bring balance in our body. Going back to yin and yang we can say that our body is in a constant state of imbalance, where yang is stronger than yin and therefore creates a continuous state of inflammation in our tissues. In other words, our sympathetic nervous system is in a constant state of alertness and keeps triggering defensive reactions of the brain. This cannot go on forever and we simply have to restore balance.

By being our own doctor we can greatly reduce the intake of toxic materials and introduce more rest and relaxation in our lives. We can start to meditate and make some changes in our lifestyle. Then there will be more balance between yang and yin and less reason for our body to be on guard all the time.

12. Less Shock Effect On Our Body

Our bodies like balance, as we already know, and they also like things to go slowly. Everything in our body goes slowly. Lets have a look: after conception it takes about 9 months for the little peanut to develop into a baby, after birth it takes about 20 years to learn what it is all about, then it takes about 50 years to live and play with the things we learned and in the meantime learn a lot more and then it takes about 20 years to slow down and eventually die. All our systems and processes are built and organised around this principle. In my opinion we should look at healthcare as a module that fits in this process. But unfortunately, healthcare is developing into a fast paced, never resting thing that does not have time to wait and see the results of its work. Medication and drugs are heavy stuff that chemically hit us over the head. They make changes in our body in a drastic way, because they bring our body chemically out of balance. The same thing goes for surgery. It always amazes me how much surgery has become, almost casually, a major part of health care and how often it is prescribed. It is obvious, of course, that surgery can be life saving and one of the great goods of modern medicine, but it should be channelled more and only performed if there is absolutely no other way out.

Surgery is literally an attack on the integrity of our body. It cuts in our flesh, creates scar tissue and leaves our body in mayhem. We almost always underestimate the time and energy we need to recover from it. Scar tissue deep down in the body interrupts – according to Chinese Medicine – the energy flow and it takes a long time for the body to find a way around it.

I call this sledgehammer therapy. It is not in balance with our body and disturbs everything greatly. If we can find a way to offer necessary changes to our body slowly and patiently, the healing process will be so much smoother and the results so much better. The problem is that we already accept surgery for certain conditions as the only way out and prepare for the long healing time. There are many situations that can be solved differently if we have the patience to let our body heal.

The way our medical system is set up leads to more drug use and surgery. It is a network of specialisations and each and every one of the participants has spent years and lots of dollars to get where they are now. So it is only logical that they want to earn as many dollars as possible back. So the general practitioner, as gatekeeper of our healthcare system, will make an assessment and often is inclined to prescribe medication. If that does not do the trick, he can refer to another health care worker, a specialist. Every practitioner wants to utilize his professional skills. I, as a physiotherapist and acupuncturist, experience the same feeling. When somebody comes in and asks if acupuncture will be effective for a certain condition, I almost always say yes. I might explain that certain situations are more tedious to treat and will take more time with uncertain chance of success, but I seldom send somebody away. The same thing goes for the chiropractor, the surgeon and any other health care practitioner. We believe in our system and we do what we do. The difference is that acupuncture is just the insertion of small needles with the intention of stimulating the body to heal and does not do any harm if it does not work, while chiropractors make mechanical adjustments, already a more forceful intrusion and surgeons cut us open, about the most disturbing thing a patient can go through. If the surgery does not work, we still have the side- and aftereffects of the procedure and have to go through the healing process, with physical and mental scar tissue.

Here are some examples. When I worked in Europe for almost 20 years in the eighties and nineties– and please forget about all the euphoric ideas people have about that continent, it is just to show some differences – carpal tunnel syndrome, nerve entrapment in the wrist, was a relatively rare condition. As soon as I started working in Canada I was surprised about all the people with that diagnose and I was even more surprised how many people went for surgery for it. Many times I have seen that complaints that might point to carpal tunnel syndrome, were the result of a wrong working posture, prolonged sitting, inactive lifestyle, computer work and so on. Many times I have seen, that by making people aware of this and by teaching them a proper working posture and giving them the right exercises the problem went away. Many times I have seen that people who underwent surgery, but did not change their ways, did not see any improvement afterwards. Of course there are people who really have a confined space in the wrist that creates carpal tunnel syndrome and who need surgery, but in my experience that is a minority.

This is an example of an expensive, often unnecessary medical procedure that can leave the patient in limbo and is often initiated based on the medical specialisation of the practitioner, while not giving other, milder options enough chance.

Another example is back surgery. Our spine is built up out of 24 movable vertebrae, 7 for the neck, 12 or the chest and 5 for the lower back. The spine is shaped like an S and during our movements all these segments work together. Because of the way we are built, standing like a pencil on its eraser, we are not very stabile, and a lot of forces are being sent through the different sections of the spine. Therefore certain areas are more prone to injury, like the lower back and the neck. Lower back pain is a major reason for people to visit a doctor. So we start focusing on the lower back, because that is where we look with our specialised eyes and that is also what the patient complains about. A typical case of a patient with lower back pain looks like this: the doctor prescribes a painkiller, if that does not help an X-ray is taken, then a referral to the physiotherapist. If exercises and local therapy don't help the patient goes back to the doctor and is referred to a specialist, usually an orthopaedic surgeon. The surgeon will do some testing and screening and, being a surgeon, chances are that he advises surgery. The lower back is one of our most sensitive areas, because of our upright posture and the way we use it. Our body is under a continuous attack of stress, day in, day out, and all that stress needs to go somewhere. We all have weak lower backs in common. Our body is always looking for a place to ventilate the stress it is under and what would be a better spot than a weak spot? So, it turns out that a lot of lower back pain is based on emotional factors that our body in some way channels to that area.

The lower back is also a major tool in doing our daily physical chores. Bending over, picking up stuff, reaching out, rotating and many times while carrying heavy loads. Because the majority of people with a physical job don't have a lot of body awareness, they use their backs in a wrong way, using it as a lever, without bending the knees enough. They also make these movements over and over again and bodies don't like repetitive movements; they always lead to injury.

So here are two major reasons for lower back pain. Obviously the patient needs to be made aware of this and be instructed how to do it better. The only way of doing this is by involving the patient in his own healing process. Passive measures like the use of physical therapy modalities, chiropractic adjustments, massages and surgery, for that matter, are not a long-term solution.

We have to make absolutely sure that everything has been tried before we send the patient for surgery. And many times that is not the case.

Before we shock body and mind with drastic procedures we should explore alternative solutions and we will be surprised how much can be fixed without the sledgehammer.

13. *Less Stress Related Issues*

When I say addictions, diabetes, fibromyalgia, hypertension, acid reflux, cholesterol, overweight, depression, dementia and cancer, what is our first reaction? Very likely we know someone in our circle of friends or family who is suffering from at least one of them. It is obvious that these are all very common health problems these days. They seem to become more frequent with an alarming rate.

I have chosen these diseases, because they are so immensely common and so many people are taking drugs to fight them. These diseases basically mirror what is going on in our society. There are many more health issues that match these criteria, but I would like to concentrate on these.

The attentive reader will already have detected the common factor in all of them. All these health problems are getting worse under stress or are even caused by stress. Let us have a look at them one by one.

Addictions. We become addicted to something when it gives us pleasure. Things that give us pleasure are drugs – so they say -, alcohol, sex, food, nicotine and so on. Then we remember the pleasure and we want more. Then, in order to experience the same amount of pleasure, we need to take more than in the beginning, because we are already getting used to it. We experience pleasure, because these activities stimulate the release of dopamine into certain areas of the brain.

Factors that can be determining in the development of an addiction are boredom, feeling of uselessness, no fulfillment in life, not having a purpose and stress.

Stress stimulates people to look for ways of relaxation and we can find that relaxation, as a quick fix, in the use of nicotine, drinking alcohol, using drugs and having sex. So stress, indirectly, increases the risk to become addicted.

There are all kinds of therapies that can help addicts to get out of the grip of the substance they are addicted to. One of the things is to try to concentrate on other, less harmful, ways of finding pleasure in life. That can be for example, learning a skill and enjoying the satisfaction it gives to accomplish something. This is a natural way of rewarding us for our efforts, instead of the easy fix of substances. It takes more time, but in the end it is longer lasting and less damaging to our health.

Another way can be concentrating on a sport and trying to become good at it.

All these things are positive influences and create a sense of freedom, independence, satisfaction and responsibility. Yes, a feeling of responsibility can be very rewarding, because it increases our self-esteem and sense of appreciation and those are basic needs in a human being.

Diabetes. When we have diabetes the body either does not produce the hormone insulin via the pancreas (type 1) or the body is resistant to its own insulin (type 2). In both cases the blood sugar level goes up and sugar is not going to the cells to provide energy. General causes for diabetes are genetic and environmental factors. Diabetes also has a lot to do with being overweight.
Stress can lead to diabetes, because under stress the body produces more stress hormone like cortisol and adrenaline. The purpose of these chemicals is to prepare the body for a survival reaction, to dodge the danger. They do that by raising the blood sugar level, to make the body produce more energy for the cells.

Fibromyalgia. This disease under this name was first mentioned in 1976, but overtime people have been suffering from conditions with similar symptoms. For a long time it was believed that it was a psychological problem and although there is now more and more proof that it is a realistic physical concern, there are still health care practitioners who believe that it is more 'between the ears'. The most important symptoms of fibromyalgia are tiredness, exhaustion, insomnia, widespread muscle pain, depression and irritable bowel syndrome.
The pain is there all the time and even at night there is no escape. So patients become more and more exhausted and because they have to fight the pain all the time, they also become depressed.
There are several causes of fibromyalgia. Basically anything that brings the central nervous system out of balance can eventually cause fibromyalgia. So, of course a lot of things that are going on in our hectic lives can be responsible, like

pollution, financial troubles or worry. The weather and atmospheric pressure can also have an effect on the severity of fibromyalgia, but the factor that has most influence is stress. Stress is something that has an effect on the whole body and fibromyalgia also affects the whole body. Stress causes our nervous system to be more on edge and the outcome can be a flare-up of fibromyalgia.

Hypertension or high blood pressure. It is hard to believe how many people are having a high blood pressure. According to the Centers for Disease Control and Prevention (CDC) 31% of Americans have high blood pressure, 1 in every 3 adults. And 1 in 3 American adults have blood pressure numbers that are higher than normal and many people with high blood pressure (47%) are not in control of their condition. Those are staggering numbers. Of course, because of these numbers, the pharmaceutical industry is doing big business. It is almost as if everyone over 30 is taking one or more kinds of medication to lower their blood pressure.
The reasons why so many people are dealing with this problem are manifold. Think about being overweight, not being physically active enough, eating a wrong diet, especially taking too much salt, drinking (too much) alcohol, smoking, worrying about everything and last but not least stress. Again, stress is the major cause of high blood pressure.
I remember when I grew up in Europe that the rules for blood pressure were different. The diastolic pressure would have to be below 100 and the systolic pressure was 100 plus your age, as a rule of thumb. So for a 50 year old, a blood pressure of 90 over 150 was not abnormal. For some reason the rules have changed, because that particular pressure would now be a stage 1 hypertension and a possible reason to prescribe medication.

Of course we live more hyper lifestyles than 40 years ago, but I cannot help but wonder why what was ok then now all of a sudden is a reason for drugs. Is that not mainly in favour of the pharmaceutical industry?

Acid reflux. Also called GERD for Gastro Esophageal Reflux Disease. Another health condition that so many people are suffering from. Stomach acid is irritating the separation between stomach and oesophagus. Diet is the main reason for this affliction, especially greasy and spicy food, coffee, sugars and alcohol. It gets worse when these foods are eaten right before going to bed. In Chinese medicine they say that the stomach energy is going in the wrong direction. It is rebelling. If the stomach is not able to digest the food properly it backs up and goes in the wrong direction leading to reflux, nausea and possibly vomiting. Although this is an ancient explanation it still makes sense. If we eat better food and not late at night there is no reason for stomach acid to act up.
Again stress is a powerfully stimulating factor to get acid reflux. Stress increases the production of cortisol, a stress hormone. As a result our digestion and immune system go down and it becomes difficult to fight inflammation. Because that is what is going on: the opening to the oesophagus is inflamed.

Cholesterol. If stress is making us angry and hostile and socially isolated it raises the level of bad cholesterol. This can be a long-term effect. Stress is a natural reaction of the body to prepare it for defence. If that is not necessary, the stress hormones stay unused and stimulate the formation of fat tissue, together with unused sugars. That is a reason for inflammation to go up.
Stress is a major reason for the formation of bad cholesterol.

Overweight. Overweight can be caused by many reasons. Examples are bad eating habits and lifestyle, genetic reasons, family disposition, low self-esteem, emotional concerns, trauma, alcohol, medications, anxiety, depression and of course stress.

As explained above, stress indirectly leads to the formation of fat tissue. Fat cells attract toxic materials and are therefore hard to break down. That makes losing weight so much harder.

Depression. Depression is one of the sad health concerns that are the result of our modern, hectic lifestyle. Life's expectations are out of proportion sometimes. We are constantly trying to satisfy what everybody wants and expects from us. We need to look nice, be assertive and intelligent, have a job with meaning and a house with standing. We need to make money to pay for all that and we hardly ever have time to be our self. If we cannot meet with all those demands it is easy to become depressed. So again, stress of everyday life is the main culprit for depression. Stress leads to the production of cortisol and adrenaline, both stress hormones, and as a result our levels of serotonin and dopamine are going down. Those are chemicals we need to be happy and experience pleasure. If we have a balanced level of serotonin and dopamine we sleep well, we have a normal appetite and sex drive, we have enough energy and stabile moods and emotions. If stress remains, it leads to depression and from there to a downward spiral.

Dementia. This is another sad problem that is also very sensitive to stress. Stress makes the level of inflammation in our body go up, in all tissues. If there is enough inflammation going on in brain tissue it can lead to structural brain damage. Researchers believe that this can also be an explanation in the occurrence of Parkinson's disease and multiple sclerosis and other neurological problems.

Cancer. Stress can be responsible for cancer in different ways. If we are under continuous stress it will eventually lower our immune system. If that is the case it is hard to fight any kind of disease. It also means that we cannot kill cancer cells. In this way stress contributes directly to the existence of cancer.
Continuous stress can also be a cause for an unhealthy lifestyle. It can lead to smoking and drinking alcohol, eating an unhealthy diet and not doing enough exercise. All that together can be a cause of cancer. In this way stress contributes indirectly to the existence of cancer.

These are all diseases that are as common as daylight and they are all either caused by stress or getting worse under stress. We need to take matters in our own hands. Going to a doctor is leaving the problem in somebody else's hands. Too many times it ends up with prescriptions, screenings, tests and hospital visits and that is definitely not bringing the stress level down. By recognizing what is going on and accepting the stress level in our bodies, we automatically start the healing process. There are countless things to do, even if some stressors are not so easily removed. Meditation, relaxation, listening to music, exercising, yoga and changing diet are just a few, that can calm our body down and slowly open the door for more awareness and confidence in what we can do. We just have to learn and trust that there is so much we can do our self to make it better. Being our own doctor can be a great help in preventing these dangerous health concerns to become a threat to us.

14. Being Our Own Doctor Benefits Our Total Being

We are not just a body. We are just as much a mind, a lot of emotions and very much a social being. We can only become a complete human being, when all these ingredients are mixed together. In our world of specialisation, we love to tear everything apart. Although the phrase 'mens sana in corpore sano, a healthy mind in a healthy body' comes from a Roman poet about two thousand years ago and although everybody we talk to, agrees that we are more than just a body, in medical science and practise there is still a very strong tendency to stick to the physical part. For example if we read about a new scientific development, a new drug, a new way of performing surgery or some form of technological advancement, it is always about the effect it will have on the body. We still don't really know how to deal with the mind, with emotions and the human psyche. If a patient goes to the doctor with a vague complaint, the first thing the doctor will do is tests and when all comes back negative, he might say that emotional factors are playing a role, but from there the road to healing is blurry.

Clear complaints are complaints like broken bones, infections, lacerations, muscle-, tendon- and joint issues like tendonitis, arthritis and neurological problems like paralysis, nerve pains etc. As soon as the autonomic nervous system gets involved, - remember the nervous system that controls everything we cannot control our self and the only thing that we can control is our movements and not even all of them -, complaints become vague. A headache for example, if it is not clearly based on a trauma to the head or a tension headache, can already become a problem. Just think about the years of research scientist have spent to understand the physiological reasons of migraine headaches. There is still no consensus, let alone what the influence of the mind can be on the existence of migraines.

I had a neighbour once who was a neurologist and he spent his whole working life doing research into migraines and did not come with a real revelation.

There is medication for migraine headaches, but all of them belong to the category of sledgehammer therapy. Some throw a blanket over the headache, but the patient still feels the presence of it underneath. Some suppress the headache, but at the same time open the door for the next attack. Some drugs are principally for something totally different, like nausea and vomiting, but have shown to also reduce a migraine headache. So it is a bit all over the place and this is just about headache. What about all the other vague complaints? How about insomnia, tiredness, circulation problems, itch, skin diseases, digestive disorders, dizziness, allergies, alternating and inconsistent pains and so on?

The autonomic nervous system with its two parts, sympathetic and parasympathetic, yang and yin if you will, reacts very strong on stress factors of all origin. It is the most important nervous system that we have, because it controls so much in our body. Stress factors attack the integrity of our body and will sooner or later have an effect on this nervous system. There is a strong link between the autonomic nervous system and our emotions. Fear, as a strong emotion, activates the sympathetic part of the system and melancholy does the opposite, by activating the parasympathetic part and making us more prone to depression. Does the stressor activate the brain to experience fear and then sets off the sympathetic reaction or is it the other way around: does the stressor activate the sympathetic nerves and the brain registers fear? Important is that there cannot be a separation between body and mind. As long as we don't give as much attention to the mind as we give to the body there will never be balance and there will always be new diseases, new ways for the body to express and ventilate the effects of stress.

It is only logical to believe that humans are not meant to be under constant negative stress. There is too much input, constantly, and that makes us sick. If we keep feeding our body with wrong food it becomes overweight, because the calories have to go somewhere. If we keep feeding our mind with negative stress it will find multiple ways to ventilate and that leads to all those vague complaints.

By understanding this principle and trying to be our own doctor we can balance between body and mind. The answers are within all of us, we can feel them if we open up for it.

15. Longevity – But Not Forever

The eternal quest to the fountain of youth still continues and if we cannot find that fountain then maybe another one that stretches life until it is thin. We certainly do not accept life as it comes, because there is always something to change or add or improve.

Again, here the main problem is stress. We are in a constant fight against the effects of stress. People who become very, very old in this world usually have one factor in common: somehow they managed to get away from stress. Maybe they did that in an early stage of their life or maybe later, but it affected their lifespan.

There was an interesting article years ago in National Geographic magazine about old people. They said that there are a couple of places in the world where people become extremely old and those places had a lot in common. They all were high in the mountains, with fresh air, they all had an ideal mix of humidity and temperature, and the people who became very old were all born in that area and never moved away. They knew each other, did hard physical work every day until a high age, drank mostly spring water or teas from the area. All they ate was from the land they lived on.

But the most important thing was that they hardly knew stress. There was no television, so they could not follow the news, they were mostly self-supporting, so they did not have to meet other people and stay away from their stress. Many of these people were far over 100 years old and many could not remember their year of birth. I remember a picture of a 99-year-old man, working the land every day with simple tools and bathing in ice-cold water.

So, that is the way to do it. Unfortunately, there are not many people anymore who can live like that. We are all caught in the ongoing rat race and while running we try to patch things up with Botox and yoga, with yoghurt and tofu and quick, orchestrated, 'relaxing' vacations. One hour of yoga per week does not do much to counter the stress of the rest of the week.

Being our own doctor means that we are constantly monitoring our self. We are becoming aware of what is going on in our body and we learn to react fast. We recognize signs and symptoms and learn what to do about it. So, that way we can lower the level of stress permanently and add some years to our life. Already we can see that happening. People are becoming older and 90 years is not an exception anymore.

16. We Know Our Own Body Best

Health care practitioners make a diagnosis, based on the symptoms that we mention and based on the signs that the body shows. What we tell is never exactly what we feel, because it is almost impossible to verbalize feelings. So we give a verbal version of what we feel and the practitioner translates that into his version. So in the end he has a picture that might be totally different from what we feel. Doing an assessment and taking a history requires a lot of listening and checking if you got it right. For example, when a person is in pain, he needs to explain what kind of pain, where, is it there all the time or interrupted and with what frequency. We can talk forever about pain and all its qualities, deep, superficial, shooting, nagging, sharp, stabbing and so on. We can all recognize the severity of pain and we can feel if it is deep or superficial, chronic or acute. We can feel the changes in pain and we can say if those changes are because of therapy or drugs or maybe because the body is trying to heal.

Of course, a therapist is totally depending on what we tell him. Because even if there are objective signs, like blood test results, X-rays, lab tests etc., what the patient experiences does not have to correspond with those results. Well known is the fact that X-rays can put us on the wrong foot. Talking about back pain, sometimes people with bad X-rays have hardly any complaints and sometimes the X-rays are not that bad, but the patient has lots of complaints. This can also be the case with blood tests or MRI scans. We cannot always diagnose just based on objective data.

We need to learn to recognise our body, what it tends to do. The more we listen to our body and open up, the more we learn. We can learn, for example, how our body reacts on certain kinds of stimuli. Migraine patients are very good at that. They usually know exactly what triggers an attack. They know this, because they have to deal with it so many times, that they have learned to listen and pay attention. The more we listen the more we learn and the more we recognize. Women are most of the time better in this than men. Women are more focused on and familiar with feelings and emotions anyway. Women tend to trust their intuition and are usually right. They are also very good at verbalizing that intuitive feeling, so, in my experience, it is always easier to find out what is wrong with a woman than with a man. Men have some kind of inborn problem to explore their feelings. It is not cool and it does not serve their immediate purpose. Men's purpose is to provide and defend and they really have no time for emotions. When men get older they become very emotional, sometimes even stronger than women. Maybe that is because the necessity to provide and defend is not so strong anymore and now the feelings come floating to the surface.

I remember giving relaxation therapy in my clinic in the Netherlands. It was a therapy where the patient had to lie down, close the eyes and start concentrating on his own body. He had to block everything else, like business, phone calls, appointments, deals, lunches and fights with his wife, you name it. Luckily this was the era just before the cell phone, so we did not have to deal with the problem of cell phone addiction.

I treated quite some businessmen, who, unwittingly, developed hyperventilation syndrome, while totally being absorbed in financial transactions.

That was of course a problem, because all of a sudden they started to sweat, couldn't concentrate anymore, were experiencing tingling sensations in the arms, becoming dizzy and confused. You really cannot have that in the middle of an important business transaction. Medication did not really work, because it was all caused by too much stress. The only way out was to recognize that and fight the stress from the inside out. I was using a very organised system, so that, at least, appealed a little bit to their rational brain. In a few weeks they could develop a technique to relax themselves in almost any given situation and once that level was reached they started to appreciate the value of relaxation, and, most importantly, they learned to listen to their own body and recognize signs and symptoms and the fact that they could do something about it.

There are also many examples of people who visit practitioners on a weekly basis for years. This is called a maintenance program. I am not really sure what is being maintained, the patients well being or the practitioners wallet. I am sure that anybody who is going through such a treatment, somewhere feels, if he opens up to it, that it is not really going anywhere. We need to feel that a treatment is stimulating and directed to a certain goal, like independence and if that is not happening we have to stop. I saw a young patient who injured his knee about 10 years ago during work. Surgery was performed to cleanout debris from the knee and physiotherapy followed for quite some time. Then, 5 years later, he injured the same knee again, because after the first time the knee never fully recovered. Again surgery was performed, followed by physiotherapy. A stabilizing brace was prescribed as well. Physiotherapy was concentrated on strengthening exercises. Recently the knee acted up for the third time. When the patient appeared for physiotherapy I really did not want to start doing all the exercises again. That had been done for almost 10 years. It was time to teach the patient to concentrate on function like walking, swimming, running, cycling etc. No more exercises. The patient was so relieved that he did not have to go through all the therapy again, but that he could now focus on something he needed in everyday life. He needed confidence and stimulation and above all balance in his life, whatever the knee decided to do.

If this patient had listened to himself and his body he would probably have decided years ago already that he needed change and a more functional approach. But, unfortunately, the system does not work like that and keeps putting people in the same routine, even if there are all kinds of signs that it is not working.

By learning to be our own doctor we can prevent such situations and cut treatment short.

Life is a game and we all play our roles. But underneath our roles is the bare human being, with emotions and feelings. So, in the end, we can all learn self-awareness, it is just a matter of training.

When we train to feel our body and trust our instincts, it becomes obvious that there are a lot of advantages connected to it.

17. Guiding The Doctor Into What We Want

I think that we are leaving our health too much in somebody else's hands. If we are lucky enough to live in the developed world we are part of the era of information, of learning, of assertiveness and of not just accepting everything. It is also the era of democracies and having a say in politics and decision-making. If we don't like what we are seeing we can decide to move away and go somewhere where we believe it is better. There is usually more money available than 50 years ago and we know our rights, so a lot of ingredients to live an independent, self-chosen life are there. So why is it that we don't show that involvement when it comes to maintaining our health? Is that because we don't know enough about it? Sure, there can be circumstances that require a more in-depth knowledge of health, but aren't we keen enough to figure that out and leave it to the professionals? If we see a doctor, we should do it in a well-founded, substantiated way. Don't forget that it is all about our health, so we want to guide the doctor and his knowledge into a direction that is beneficial to us. That is also what health-care is supposed to be. It is a store where we buy health and pay for it, through tax dollars and insurance premiums and it is definitely not cheap. So we have to try to get what we want and not what the system wants. Years ago it was the doctor who decided what was going to happen and we just followed, but that was then. I know that people are slowly waking up, but there are still too many of us who just follow and not think.

I also had the tendency, especially in the beginning, to guide the patient in a direction that I had chosen. And most of the time that was ok and no questions asked. But slowly I realised that it was not about me, but about the patient and that I had to listen and look and try to find out what he wanted.

The secret of proper health care is giving the patient what he wants and that is only possible if we listen and learn.

Health care practitioners can be very strong in their beliefs what is good for the patient. The way we approach a patient is depending on so many factors, like education, experience, religion, upbringing, culture etc. All these things make a human being who he is, and if that human being happens to work with patients he will without any doubt project his background on the patient. And that is wrong, because the patient is not really interested in the doctor's background. He wants to get better.

People's bodies and minds don't want to be sick, they want to be in balance. The only way of reaching that is by finding what that particular patients balance is.

I have this older gentleman as a patient. He is close to eighty and has a degree in biochemistry. His mind is formed by what he has been studying his whole life, very analytical, very detailed, very exact. That is how he thinks, he does not know any other way. I always ask my patients if they are ok if I give them some acupuncture and 99% says yes. Not this gentleman, he is not interested, cannot get his head around it. Although that is fine and his choice, I cannot help feeling a little bit disturbed, because it is my thing, how can he reject my thing? But I have learned over the years that I have to let go of that and adjust to what the patient wants. I am now treating him with physiotherapy modalities and I try to explain everything as clear and logical as possible and he is happy and improving.

So, this is a patient who knows what he wants and who is not afraid of sending me the message and that is how it should be. He tells me where he wants my help and expertise and I comply, even if I think that he might do a lot better if he would let me do it my way. If we buy a car, we go to the dealership, tell the sales rep what car, what color and what bells and whistles, whether he likes it or not. That is a normal thing to do and everyone accepts it. We should do the same thing with our health. Before going to the doctor, we should do our due diligence. Read about the problem, try to do our own diagnosis and write down questions, about things that are not clear. That way we seem determined, gain self esteem, show the doctor that we want to be involved, but at the same time are open for advice. We might irritate the doctor to no end, but so be it. It is our health, and by the time we leave the office he is concentrating on somebody else and probably forgot about us.

We have to guide the doctor instead of the other way around, but be polite and open-minded and establish a mutual respectful relationship. That way we both win: the doctor feels appreciated because we ask his opinion and we feel good, because we were involved with our own problem and feel listened to.

18. Best Treatment First

By listening and learning we become more and more aware of our self and we also learn how we react best in case of sickness. We know how we react on drugs in general and whether or not we react well on herbs or alternative medicine.

Almost everybody I speak to tells me that deep down they don't want to take medication and people who don't are proud that they don't. We feel inside that the taking of drugs is not in balance with our body. There are always side effects, sometimes so strong that they make the drugs almost useless.

Not all people react like that, because it depends on what they believe. If we believe that the drug is the best solution, our body will already start to open up for it. It is guided by our mind. If people really want to be treated with drugs then they should do that, because there is a fair chance that it will help them.

I also know people who absolutely do not react well on the use of herbs or alternative medicine. This is probably so, because deep down they don't believe that it is going to help them. That is a very powerful force. It can also be that these people used to take a lot of chemical drugs and by doing so have made their body less sensitive for the relatively weak stimulus of herbs or alternative medicine. Like a patient I had recently who had been taking amitriptyline (among others used for neuropathic pain) for 15 years. He had all kinds of complaints, pain all over the body, tiredness, fibromyalgia etc., and I treated him with acupuncture, because these conditions usually react very well on acupuncture. The treatment did not seem to have much effect, which was strange, because people usually react very fast. After 3 treatments he told me about the amitriptyline and that he had decided to cut its use in half and slowly get rid of it altogether. Immediately his condition improved, he had less pain and he could handle the situation better. It turned out that the chemical working of the drug was too strong for the relatively weak stimulus of acupuncture needles to sort an effect. After he had reduced his medication intake, acupuncture was much more successful.

We also see that by concentrating on our self and listening and learning we can make our body more receptive and sensitive to herbs and alternative medicine overtime. Everything is a learning process. Another example: I developed acid reflux in the last couple of years. In the beginning I tried to deal with it with over the counter antacids. Eventually this did not work anymore. I did not make any changes in my eating habits, so the reflux stayed and got worse. I received a prescription for drugs and used this for a while. As long as I was taking these pills everyday, I was fine, but I just could not keep doing it.

I started to make changes in my eating pattern. No more coffee at night, no fatty foods, not so much sugar and no more eating after 8 pm. I felt immediately better and did not need to take the medication everyday anymore. When I needed the drug, I knew why and what I did wrong. When my wife and I did a low sugar diet for a few weeks I did not need the pills at all. I had listened to my body and learned how to make changes. I felt that I had my body more under control, a very satisfying feeling.

The same thing can happen with other kinds of medication. When our blood pressure is high, we can usually figure out why. There is always stress to reckon with and we can always make changes in our diet and lifestyle. Nobody gets high blood pressure without a reason. Our responsibility is to find that reason and eliminate it, not just start popping pills and hope for the best.

We can hone our body by being alert. And by doing so, we will be able to choose the best treatment first. That means that there will be fewer try-outs, because we can guide the doctor better. We will get less unnecessary medication in our body and fewer toxins.

19. *Fewer Treatment Protocols*

We are living in an organised world. Some countries are a bit more organised than others, but in general we are well organised. That is of course a necessity with the billions of people who live on this planet. So, organisation is everywhere and makes life liveable and manageable. That usually is a good thing, but not always, because often the organisation becomes more important than the goal. Health care is also busy organising everything, especially in big institutions like hospitals. That is why hospitals are not nice places to visit. The moment we step through the door we are caught in the system. There is no personal approach, no time and not much empathy. We must follow blue or yellow lines to far away departments and wait in impersonal waiting rooms. The receptionist usually booked 10 to 15 minutes for us, to talk to the doctor about major concerns that greatly affect our life and that often after waiting for months or even years for an appointment. There is not much individuality and these visits easily lead to frustration and uncertainty.

The reason for this system is money of course. Health care is extremely expensive and doctors need to process many patients in minimal time.

Once the intake has been done the actual treatment has to begin. Many medical treatments these days are performed on the basis of a protocol. Protocols are precisely described programs and procedures a patient has to go through after his diagnosis has been made. There are some advantages of protocols, for example when it is used as a checklist during a first assessment. That way no important information is missed during the initial meeting with the patient.

My concern is the use of protocols in treatment. It is another way of making healthcare impersonal. Because of the multitude of patients and the high costs of the care there is already not much time to pay attention to the patient. By using protocols, yet another chance to get to know the patient is lost, because, regardless of whom the patient is, the treatment is already determined.

In secondary care institutions, like hospitals, getting around the protocols is difficult, because the system is built upon them. In primary care, there is a much more personal contact between care provider and patient and more room for letting go of the protocols.

Physiotherapy clinics are part of primary health care and used to be a personal and individual discipline, where patients were guided in their therapy in a relaxed atmosphere. Over the years more and more treatment protocols have been developed, at least for the more common health conditions. Described are the exercises, what kind and how many repetitions, what kind of physio-technical-modalities have to be used and how long the treatment is supposed to last.

In Europe, where I used to live and work, there was even a connection between the use of these treatment protocols and reimbursement of the treatment price by health care insurers in some countries.

This is of course not in the interest of the patient. It is, though, a typical sign of how patients are seen these days in Western countries. It is all very technical and very mechanical.

I can understand that very technical procedures like complicated surgeries have a protocol. The patient is unconscious and the surgeons perform a technical procedure, regardless of whom the patient is. I can also understand that after surgery, a protocol must be followed for rehabilitation, so that the wound gets a chance to heal. But there, where a more personal approach is feasible, we should let go of pre-cooked procedures and pay more attention to the individual patient.

By being our own doctor we can learn a lot about our problem and become a partner in the solution together with the practitioner and take away the need for impersonal protocol. After all, we are already actively involved.

20. Attention – We Love It

Probably what people crave most, in the middle of all those addictions, is attention.

After all, we are human beings and our most precious possession is our self. Attention confirms who we are and gives us a feeling of satisfaction and self esteem.

There is just such a big difference between living now and in our (baby boomer) time 50 years ago. We grew up a lot more modest and reserved and we were more passive and waiting for recognition by others. Applying for a job was a matter of writing a stylish letter, polite and with reservation and full of respect towards the possible future employer.

Now life is totally different. We are living in the time of I, me and myself. Social networks like Facebook, meant to share, are now more a platform to showcase one self. Everybody has a profile, with even the smallest of achievements enlarged and bolded, like they were university degrees. Pictures are presented as if the subject is coming right out of a Hollywood studio and 90% of them are selfies.

In resumes and job interviews we are all dynamic, efficient, outgoing and even aggressive. Where is the modesty and self-reflection? Once the job has been secured most of us want paycheques, but please, not so much responsibility. Attention is a wonderful thing and definitely a must for a human being. Without attention we wither away and cannot fully bloom. Modern medicine is not really an example of giving its players attention. Long-term lack of attention will make people vulnerable and eventually sick and trying to find help in a system that is notorious for its lack of attention is certainly not going to help. If we don't get attention, we are going to ask for it and what is a better way than being our own doctor? We will always give our self the most attention and that can already be a healing factor. Then, if we go to see the doctor, we can guide him in the direction that we want and assure our self of attention. I hate it if I made an appointment with a doctor and then at the promised time I have to wait. I think that my time is just as valuable as anyone else's and it does not matter whether the other party is a doctor, a lawyer or whoever. So I have a rule, that when I make an appointment with a doctor (I don't see that many lawyers luckily), I will wait 15 minutes and then I am gone. Sometimes that backfires, because now I have to make another appointment and drive there again, but most of the time it gives me a satisfied feeling and a form of pride that I have chosen for myself. And, many times, the doctor feels uncomfortable and later apologizes. So, by choosing for myself and showing the doctor that I have respect for myself and expect that back, I have won what I crave most, attention. Now my visit will be different, because suddenly I am not number 25 anymore, but the guy who walked away and left the doctor standing. I cannot understand why people are spending hours in waiting rooms, losing their self-respect and feeding the system in the process.

If you smile to others you will get a smile in return, if you are nice to people, they will be nice to you, if you show that you have self-respect you will be treated with respect. This works all the time. If we visit a store and the clerk is not interested and rude, all we need to do is ask him right there, why he is not interested and rude. That always creates a huge change. Be respectful and expect respect.

By being our own doctor we give attention to our self and by becoming aware of our body and its problems we can act self-assured and get the attention that we deserve.

21. Personable And Portable Health

I am convinced that we are all smart people. Some think that they are not, but they are, they just don't know how to use it and develop it. When there are so many people around, who all want the same thing, they start to behave like sheep; where one goes, the other goes. But that also means that they don't have to think anymore, they just follow. Following, without thinking is a bad thing, because it does nothing for our self-esteem and it does not give us the satisfaction of being creative. Unfortunately, the big masses of - often low educated - people are mainly followers and followers can be manipulated by people who know that they are smart, and before you know it we are all following the leader, who can do whatever he wants: an ancient principle of governing, even the Romans knew it: panem et circenses, give the people bread and games. In other words keep them happy and well fed and you can do what you want.

So, we have to be do-ers, not followers, or even better, leaders. As soon as we become creative, we become leaders. That is definitely the case with trying to be our own doctor. The training and self-awareness make the experience personable. We are now forced to think for our selves and come up with a solution. We become more alert of things that might be going on. We develop a kind of sensitivity for our state of health and can react fast. Like a doctor, we can now carry our own little bag with tools and enjoy portable health.

22. Knowing The Difference Between Chronic And Acute Problems

An acute illness usually starts suddenly and the pain is sharp in quality. Change happens fast. Most of the time acute illnesses disappear again without too much intervention. Chronic illnesses have been there for a long time and don't disappear on their own. The pain is more vague and nagging. Many times an acute disorder that has not been treated well can turn into a chronic problem. When an acute disorder is the result of a trauma, a fracture or surgery, modern medicine can be extremely effective. Alternative medicine can also be effective in the treatment of acute problems, like the application of acupuncture for acute pain.

Chronic disorders are a whole different problem. They are harder to treat and are far more costly. The major factor that makes health care almost unaffordable is the treatment of chronic complaints. People who are suffering from chronic pain, for example, keep coming back into the system.

Of course everything happens with a reason and we don't just get a sickness out of nothing. A lot of chronic conditions have a relationship with our life. They react on what we eat, how we sleep, whether we are emotionally stabile etc. So indirectly, chronic problems are connected with stress, tension, emotions, diet and so on.

We already knew that these ingredients could make us sick. In order to find a solution, we need to start self-exploration. That means monitoring our self and recognizing symptoms. Trying to be our own doctor.

If people have been suffering from a chronic disease they sometimes lose their believe in themselves. They don't believe that they can get better. Getting better often means sacrificing things, like lifestyle, diet, habits, money etc. It is not always so easy to make those choices. Sometimes making changes costs money and a lot of people are afraid of change. But once we know what the benefits can be it can suddenly become very interesting. There might be a chance to reduce or get rid of the long-term use of medication. And when that happens our body slowly starts to become more active and starts to take over and creates more balance. With many chronic complaints the autonomic nervous system is involved.

This is the modern version of what the ancients called yin and yang, the battlefield of balance. Headache, insomnia, tiredness, undefined pain, digestive disorders, dizziness, tinnitus, concentration disorders, depression, worry, allergies and asthma are all typical examples of chronic complaints.

23. Weak Spots – Everybody Has Them

This is a phenomenon that has always intrigued me. A good example that people are individuals and deserve to be treated like that is the existence of weak spots. Everybody has weak spots. For some it can be their stomach, for others it can be their head. Other examples of well-known weak spots are lower back, neck, lungs, heart, throat and muscles/tendons.

Having a weak spot means that every time something happens with our state of health or every time when we become tired and overdo it and our resistance goes down, the weak spot will show itself first. We can compare weak spots with ventilation openings in the body, so that when the pressure becomes too high it can blow off steam, like volcanoes in the earth's crust.

A very good example is the head. Many people have their head as a weak spot. They can get headaches every time when something is out of balance. These headaches can have very clear reasons, like women developing migraines before, during or after their period. Those are headaches based on hormonal imbalances. Other clear reasons are stress and emotions that can lead to tension headaches. But for those people a headache can also start when they have flu or when they did not sleep well or when they are very tired. Any imbalance can lead to a headache. Having the head as a weak spot means that also other areas of the head can be involved. Many people react on imbalances with toothache, sinus infections, earache, tinnitus, sensitive eyes, blurry vision or facial paralysis or -pain.

The lower back is another major area of weakness, perhaps even the biggest. About 75% of lower back pain complaints have an emotional connection. So stress, expectations, pressure and lack of appreciation can all lead to lower back pain. And that is apart from all the physical reasons. If the back is a weak spot it can be a constant reason of concern. The same thing goes for the neck. Muscle tensions tend to go to the neck and shoulder area. People say: I tend to carry my stress in my neck and shoulders. They already confirm the existence of a weak spot.

Areas like the head and the lower back are very common weak spots and many people will recognize that. But there are also more rare areas, typical for a certain individual. The throat can be one, for example. People with weak throats can have a constant build-up of phlegm in the throat and need to clean it all the time. Their voice can be raspy and they will definitely not become great singers. When they go outside in the cold they have to be careful not to catch a cold and protect their throat against wind and draft. Other people will have a tendency to develop all kinds of tendon inflammations. They easily get a tennis elbow or a golfers elbow, or a shoulder tendonitis. They have a very high basic tension in their muscles and there is always a lot of pull on the tendons. Others again have to deal with muscle cramps. Whenever there is a change in their diet they get cramps. It can be a low blood sugar level or a high one or a lack of calcium, magnesium and potassium. But general tiredness can also lead to muscle cramps. It is not always simple to find a logical explanation, except that the area is someone's personal weak spot.

Weak spots can also develop after an injury or surgery. An injury near muscles and joints can make that area weak. Injuries often lead to the formation of scar tissue and therefore to a lack of blood circulation.
I remember a man with a dislocation of his collarbone, where it meets the shoulder blade. It was swollen and painful. During the treatment he got a flu infection and his resistance went down. The body wanted to get rid of toxic material and chose the area of the injured joint to do that. He developed an ulcer right on top of the joint. That joint was at that moment the weakest spot in his body, so an easy choice to vent.
Sport injuries can also easily lead to the development of weak spots. Somebody who plays tennis, for example, and tries to return a difficult ball, can suddenly pull a muscle in the calf. It feels like that same tennis ball hit you in the calf. It usually heals fast, because it is pure muscle tissue with lots of blood supply, but at the same time it creates a weak

spot and the same area can easily tear again. Soccer players who are being tackled over and over again develop weak spots in their knees to a point where surgery is necessary and from then on a permanent weak spot has been created. Runners can get muscle spasms, cramps and tears in their hamstrings and will always be bothered by it, whenever they perform.

When people have a serious health condition that compromises their immune system, several weak spots can act up at the same time. Just look at cancer patients who have to undergo chemotherapy. Chemotherapy will always target certain areas with everyone, like blood cells and hair growth, but someone's weak spots will always be involved. Weak spots are very individual and only the patient knows where they are and how they tend to react on different kinds of strain. Here is another reason for us to be our own doctor. We can act proactively and concentrate from the beginning on the right areas of our body.

24. Diagnoses and stickers

The established medical world is built upon the making of diagnoses. Countless hours and tests are spent to find a diagnosis. Once the diagnosis is found it becomes a sticker on our forehead. And once the sticker is there we start behaving accordingly. When the sticker says migraine headache, our behaviour will be like this:

We are careful with noises and bright light
We don't want too much touching and moving around
We like rest and quiet
We don't like heavy physical activity
We don't like stress
We don't want to go out

We really like to be left alone

When the sticker says acid reflux disease, our behaviour
will be like this:

We don't want to eat greasy food
We don't want to eat spicy food
We don't want to eat late at night before bedtime
We don't want to drink too much coffee
We don't want to eat too many sweets

When the sticker says allergies, our behaviour can be like
this:

We don't want to be close to pets
We don't want to walk between blooming trees
We don't want to eat dairy products
We don't want to eat peanuts

All these are legitimate symptoms that belong to the
mentioned diagnosis. The problem is that after the
diagnosis has been made we no longer behave freely,
because we automatically embed the symptoms and
prognosis in our lifestyle. That is the problem, because all of
a sudden we no longer are who we always have been, we
are now somebody with a sticker. Other people can see the
sticker and adjust their behaviour towards us and we can
adjust our behaviour towards others. That is not right of
course, because in the end we still are who we are.
What is really going on in the body is something that we
don't want or find difficult to address. Whether we are
suffering from migraine headaches, acid reflux disease or
allergies, they themselves are all symptoms of an imbalance
in our body. And most of the time that imbalance is a
reduced immune system and way too many toxins inside.

The body has to work so hard to expel the toxins that eventually it's immune system suffers and we get sick. That is where we have to focus and not on the stickers.

Of course I am telling you nothing new. We all know that modern medicine is often occupied with fighting symptoms. We also know that once the symptoms are suppressed, but nothing basically changes, they will come back or need to stay suppressed by drugs.

Half a century ago, when people were not so involved with their health, this was normal procedure that not many questioned and the occasional ones that did were mostly seen as weird. But now there is so much more awareness about health and so much more willingness to change and keep our self in good order, that it is amazing that we are still following the same guidelines. Why do we not change? Why is there not more money available for research in to alternative, but better approaches to health? The answer is probably twofold. First of all more than half the money made available for medical research is coming from the pharmaceutical industry, and they are not really interested in helping to develop the competition. The second reason is that many people just don't want to change, because they are happy with the pill. They believe in the pill and thus it works. Life is a matter of perception: the truth is the way we see it. If we are raised with the pill, then that is our truth and the older we get, the harder it is to perceive another truth.

But if, after many conventional interventions from medication to drugs and many diagnoses, the patient does not see a positive outcome, he may start looking for something else and open up for another truth.

A 56-year old woman is diagnosed with MS, fibromyalgia, migraine headaches, swelling in the legs, digestive disorders, inflammation all over etc. She is constantly tired, not in the least from the side effects of the medication she has been taking.

The sticker MS is the brightest one on her forehead and dominates all the others. It carries so many different symptoms and it affects so many aspects of her life that it alone can already be responsible for whatever else she has been diagnosed with.

She is coming in to the clinic with as her main concern migraine headache. She also wants some core exercises, because she feels weak and does not have any energy left. I talk to her about her general state of health and soon it becomes clear that she is fed up with the medication and the ongoing tests and diagnoses. I suggest acupuncture and she accepts a try-out, because she is not totally free yet of the stickers. According to Chinese medicine she has a very clear picture that reflects all the things that she has been going through. Most important issues in het body are a weak functioning digestive system – responsible for energy and water metabolism – and a lot of heat build-up. Lack of energy makes her tired, not functioning of water metabolism creates swelling in the legs and the formation of mucus and the heat causes the widespread inflammation. All this is visible in the tongue: fiery red and swollen with a thick yellow coating and a pulse that is deep, vague, fast and slipping.

What a relief not to have to think about MS or fibromyalgia, but to just see and confirm all the symptoms that fit so neatly together in a Traditional Chinese Medicine syndrome called damp heat in the Middle Burner. When they created those syndromes thousands of years ago, they never heard of MS, because it was not invented yet and Chinese medicine only looked at the yin/yang imbalance in the body.

This patient had made a conscious choice to do something else and, after initial hesitation, opened up to a different approach. She had shifted her perception and discovered a new truth. She had become her own doctor. She now uses the benefits of both systems and manages to control her condition with less medication and more confidence in herself.

In the US there is the National Center for Complementary & Alternative Medicine (NCCAM) and in Canada there is IN-CAM Research network. They perform research on complementary and alternative medicine, but it is, compared to conventional medicine, still small. In the end it is of course always a matter of money.
As long as sicknesses are big business, like diabetes, cancer, obesity and so on, it will always be a hard battle to try to find a real solution. Real solutions mean less business, so we don't want to put dollars in that. It is also about information given to the public. Giving information about healthy lifestyle habits and dieting – although growing - is still not mainstream and too often seen as coming from 'the soft sector'.
If we would recognize on a big scale that lifestyle, stress and eating habits are the main culprits of sickness, we would see that the stickers would be less meaningful and that we should change our ways.
If governments and industry are not contributing enough to concentrate on the real causes and solutions then we should focus again on being our own doctor. In the end the only one who is really interested in us is us. We are the only ones who can be really concerned about our health and who want to do whatever it takes to make it better. We are also the only ones who can feel what is going on and what the best solution would be eventually.
Being our own doctor is not just about monitoring our health and trying to find the best solution; it is a way of life. It represents the wish to be independent and self-

supporting, to not be afraid of change and initiative. It recognizes the value of our self-awareness in health and all kinds of other issues. It recognizes the strength of the power inside our self, the power to heal and to make changes in our circumstances. Too many of us are followers and don't even know what abilities they have inside. It is all about energy, energy to think and to act. The ancient Chinese already played with that concept, so it was obvious in those days already that it was there. For some odd reason we have wiped the concept of energy from our table. For us, everything needs to be concrete, visible and touchable and if it's not that, than it simply does not exist. We do accept energy in so many forms, electrical energy, heat energy, water energy, fossil fuel energy and so on. Something makes something else move, clear enough. Nobody thinks twice about the fact that a car moves because of the energy generated by fuel. But if we say that blood flows in the blood vessels, because of the energy generated within the body by food, drink etc., then all of a sudden it becomes mystique, religious and vague. Especially when we turn it around and say that the blood, in turn, transports the energy through the body. Without energy nothing happens in the body, why is that so hard to grasp? If we don't maintain our car and put fuel in it, it won't go, at least not for long. That is a nice, clear thought. If we don't maintain our body and we put food in it, it won't go either. Already a bit more confusing. The answer is of course, that bodies don't run only on food. They need, apart from good food and drink, a balanced mind, a stress free environment, enough activity and, above all, direction.

All these ingredients cannot be found at the doctor's office or in the hospital. They are stored in our minds and we have to slowly learn to recognize and use it.

It is a pity that so many patients decide to go a different route only at the very end of the medical road. Only after all conventional options have been exhausted and satisfaction has not been found, do we open up for the alternative. Therefore alternative approaches usually have to deal with chronic situations and a very toxoid body. Most people don't know that alternative medicine can also be very effective for acute situations and then even faster, because the problem is fresh.

Western diagnoses are very stigmatizing and leave people with a sticker on their forehead that determines their behaviour to the outside world as well as the behaviour of others towards them. Diagnoses can be paralyzing and can prevent the body from healing.
By being our own doctor we can get away from the diagnoses as much as possible and try to find an effective solution within the boundaries of our own minds.
If the sickness is so aggressive that the milder techniques of alternative medicine cannot touch it, we can always decide to go the other route.

25. Cost Control

Last but not least there is the aspect of money. We all know that health care is extremely expensive and every year governments spend more and in every election money for health care is a hot topic.
Most of us have no idea of the actual costs of health care, because we seldom see an invoice. The majority goes straight to the insurance companies.

A quick search on the Internet gives us some impressions:

According to CostHelper.com a broken leg costs up to $ 2,500, without surgery. With surgery a broken leg costs from $ 17,000 to $ 35,000. We will have to add a doctors fee between $100 and $ 2000, X-rays between $ 200 and $ 1,000 and costs for a cast around $250. This is without the rental of crutches, physiotherapy and possible hardware removal after recovery.

Pheww, just a broken leg!

Let's have a look at the costs for a colonoscopy. CostHelper.com tells us that the average price for a colonoscopy is $3,000. An ultrasound costs around $200, a vaginal delivery costs between $9,000 and $ 17,000, a C-section between $ 14,000 and $ 25,000.

Cortisone injections can cost from $25 to $ 300 per shot and flu-shots from $5 to $ 30 per shot. A visit to the emergency room can be between $ 150 and $ 3,000 and for critical care even up to $ 20,000. A visit to the doctor is around $ 90.

It is clear that many of these procedures cannot be replaced by being our own doctor. And that is exactly what the benefits of modern medicine are. If we need it it's there, but we don't always need it and that is where we save a lot of money, taxpayer's money and out-of-pocket money.

A person can develop Carpal Tunnel Syndrome based on posture, physical activities, repetitive movements etc. If we wait long enough until this becomes a real problem, a doctor might refer such a patient to a surgeon. The costs for surgical Carpal Tunnel treatment are about $7,000 per hand plus rehabilitation.

A person who is self aware and trained in monitoring himself regarding health issues, will undoubtedly know what might have caused the problem in the first place. He will know that his work is a very important factor and contributor, just as all his other daily activities. He will know if he wakes up in the morning with a stiff neck and a tingling feeling in the hand. Then he can already make a connection between these factors and the pain in the hand. Now he can go to the doctor and ask for a referral to a physiotherapist, but, to save money, he can also go to the physiotherapist directly. He can give the physiotherapist clear information about what is going on and what he thinks himself might be the problem. That can limit the amount of treatments necessary for this issue.

At a general rate of $75 for a physiotherapy treatment it is clear how much money can be saved, by being smart and self-aware. A maximum of 10 physiotherapy treatments should be more than enough to solve this problem, or a total investment of $ 750 instead of $7,000.

Another example where being our own doctor can save dollars is the problem of insomnia, or not being able to sleep. It is amazing how many people are suffering from this. Obviously, often our lifestyle and the expectations and stress our society brings with it are to blame and modern medicine has modern solutions, like a sleep study in a sleep centre to determine what kind of sleep disorder the patient has or the prescription of sleeping pills.

Sleep studies run between $1,000 and $ 3,000 and many times end up with the prescription of medication or the use of a CPAP machine. That is a machine that provides a constant flow of air to the patient through a mask. Because insomnia is such an individual problem, there can be many reasons that don't require medication or a machine.

Again a self aware patient, who is willing to have a close look at his circumstances in life, like stress levels, work pressure, financial worries, family issues, diet and so on, will undoubtedly recognise factors that can contribute to his insomnia. Instead of going straight to the doctor and possibly a sleep centre, he can decide to start doing yoga or any other relaxation therapy that appeals to him. He can make changes in his daily life, his diet and physical activity

and if nothing works he can make an appointment with a
chiropractor or another alternative health care practitioner,
like an acupuncturist to help him with balancing his
nervous system.
For $ 1,000 to $ 3,000 there are a lot of other options
available that are healthier and more focused on the
involvement of the patient into his problem.

As a final example I want to talk about a patient with jaw
pain and neck pain.
A patient who presents himself with pain in the jaws,
sometimes radiating to the neck and ears or creating a
headache is often referred to a dentist. A dentist, obviously,
will look at the patient with a dental eye and will try to
detect dental causes of this problem. It can be a
misalignment of the teeth, or a wrong occlusion, where
upper and lower teeth don't interlock with each other
properly. The dentist might prescribe orthodontic
treatment or a retainer to align the teeth with each other.
Average orthodontic treatment with braces costs about
$5,000 and retainers, if not included, run between $200 and
$1,000.
The jaw joints are very small joints that are unique in their
physiology, because they are connected to each other by the
jaw and cannot be moved separately. People have a
tendency to ventilate their worries and stress through the
head and the face. Think about the nervous ticks, tension
headaches, ear ringing, dizziness etc. Many people grind
their teeth during sleep as a reaction to stress. This is called
bruxism. Because the muscles that surround the jaw are
very strong (chewing and biting), the forces that are applied
on the jaw joints during the night, or unwittingly during the
day, are exceptional and can lead to pain and damage to the
little joints. In severe cases the pain can start to radiate to

the neck and the ears and cause neck- and ear problems and sometimes headaches.

Patients who want to be their own doctors will start monitoring themselves. They will recognise the stress they are under and will see a connection between their pain and the emotional factors of their lives. They can also feel that in the morning after waking up, their complaints are worse and the jaws feel tired. If they decide to go to the doctor they can ask pointed and focused questions and lead the doctor to, what they believe, might be the cause of the problem. The doctor might refer to a physiotherapist, because giving special exercises that help the jaw to align and reduce the spasms and grinding of the teeth, often solve the problem. These exercises can be taught in just a couple of sessions and will save a lot of money. If the exercises don't help, the patient can always visit a dentist and provide him with information about what he already has done. At the same time the patient experiences the satisfaction of having diagnosed his problems and having found a cheap and effective solution, which includes his involvement. The answer is always the education of the patient. It does not matter what kind of therapy a patient seeks, he should not be asked to come back again and again, without making him understand what is going on and what he can do about it himself. His involvement is crucial and makes him as independent as possible in the pursuit of his health. Many times pills, surgery and machines are not the long-term answer for chronic problems, because it makes people dependant and it is usually too expensive.

These are just a few examples and you would be surprised how often this happens. We can definitely make healthcare a lot cheaper by being our own doctors.

Summary

As we can see there are many advantages to being our own doctor. We should never forget that we are individuals, independently functioning organisms, and that we always get satisfaction from accomplishing something ourselves. In a world with so much stress and so many responsibilities and expectations it might look sometimes very inviting to let go and let somebody else do the thinking, but our health is too close to our wellbeing to leave it totally in the hands of others. We need to be involved and it is not always so complicated, once we have learned how to listen.

Many Times The Answers To Our Health Questions Are Not That Far Away

Chapter 6

Examples Of Being Our Own Doctor And Listening To Our Body

I just want to give two examples of health conditions that can give clear signals that point us in the right direction if we know what to look for.

Back Pain

Let us start with the back. Lower back pain is one of the most common health issues doctors and physiotherapists, chiropractors and acupuncturists have to deal with. It is a big area and affects almost everything we do. People are especially at risk when they sit a lot, like office clerks and professional drivers, or when they have to carry a lot of weight on a daily basis. The pain usually starts in the lower back and can stay there, but it can also radiate up between the shoulder blades, to the front of our body or down a leg. Sometimes, there is only pain in the heel or in the calf and nowhere else. If we don't know how to recognize our body signs we will think immediately that it is a local problem in the heel or the calf. If we go to the doctor and tell our complaints most of them will concentrate on the painful area, because that is the way they are educated. They might think of a heel spur or plantar fasciitis or maybe a pulled calf muscle. But if there is back pain in our history, either local or radiating somewhere, we must involve the back in our assessment. Very often the pain felt in heel or calf is the result of nerve irritation in the lower back and treatment should be focused there. If we are trained in listening to our body we can give the doctor useful information and get the right treatment as soon as possible.

A lot of problems in the leg are connected to the back and the nervous system. I always compare it with a garden with lots of bushes and plants. When the water supply becomes scarce, the weakest plants die first. In the leg are many weak spots, like the joints or certain muscle groups that are used intensely, so if the nerve supply and blood circulation from the lower back are involved it can easily lead to problems in those areas. So, always think about the back when you had back pain before and there is something not right in the leg.

Most of the lower back pain starts from the 4th and 5th lumbar vertebra. That is the weakest area in our lower back and that is also where most of the flexion and extension movements take place. Herniated and bulging disks with pain radiating down the back or outside of the leg are mostly located there. Another area that is weak in the lower back is a little bit higher, at the level of T12 and L1. That is the section of the spine where the round mid back changes into the hollow lower back. It is a natural transfer station and those places are always vulnerable. If there is nerve compression from that area it creates a radiating pain from the waist and via the side of the pelvis to the groin. Many times attention is focused on local tissues like gluteal muscles, SI-joints, piriformis syndrome or even the hip joint, while all the time the cause is the spine.

Of course, if a back condition exists for a longer time, these local weaknesses become a real problem, but we should never forget that the cause might very well be somewhere else and a final solution will not be found until we address that.

A 43-year-old man, good physical condition, is complaining about lower back pain for more than 10 years. The pain is always in the same location, about as big as an apple. It gets worse when riding a bicycle, something he really loves to do. He tells me that he plays drums, always sitting in a certain position. He also tells me that he has a slight scoliosis, an unnatural curve in the spine.

During the assessment it turns out that the direction of the scoliosis works directly against his preferred sitting position when he plays the drums and when he sits on his bicycle. Because these two forces work against each other, there is a constant friction that causes the pain. Assessment also shows a slight difference in leg length as a result of the scoliosis. He has a preferred sitting position, as all of us do. We all have preferences in our daily activities, based on the way our spine is built. We will automatically choose positions and posture that correspond with that preference, but if there is a force working against it, there is a problem. This is not a simple complaint to figure out. But in this case the patient was aware of his body and he knew what kind of habits he had and that really made a difference and pointed me into the right direction. The treatment is now concentrated on reducing the impact of the scoliosis and we are on the right track from the beginning. The doctor had said that he did not have to do exercises for the scoliosis, because it was just a slight one. It turned out that that was exactly the problem.

What we also need to remember in a case like this is the age factor. An otherwise healthy man of 43 is not supposed to have a recurring back pain for more than 10 years if nothing else is wrong. If somebody presents like that we should look for a more posture related cause and that is where the patient can really help.

Swollen Hands And Feet

I saw a young woman, 21 years old, slender figure, good health. She was very active in sports and very much aware of her diet, which is not always the case with 21 year-old. She was complaining about waking up in the morning with swollen feet and lower legs and sometimes with swelling in her hands. This had been going on for about 4 weeks. The doctor couldn't find anything wrong. Blood work and heart function were normal. I had treated this patient before with acupuncture for recurring headaches and slight depression. Right from the beginning the story did not make sense. Such a young and active woman should not be suffering from all these complaints, especially not because she was enjoying her life, was studying and looking forward to the new and exciting things in her life.

The acupuncture treatments for her headache worked very well and reduced the headache considerably. The treatments for the swelling also worked, but slower: first there was not much change, then she woke up without swelling in her hands since a long time, then the swelling in her hands came back, but the feet were really better. The results were erratic. That was another thing that did not make sense. Normally children and young adults react very fast on acupuncture treatments, because their bodies are young and flexible and not yet used to certain ways. This was not a reaction I had expected.

We talked and started to explore her general health to see if we could find a cause for her problems and for the fact that she did not react properly on the treatment.

Apart from an anti conceptive, she was not taking any prescription drugs. The anti conceptive she had been using for four years. The Internet told me that the side effects of this drug were, among others: headache, swelling of hands and feet and tendency to depression, all of which she had been suffering from.

Anti conceptive drugs have come a long way since they were introduced in the 1960's. But they still have an effect on the hormonal balance and some women have a hard time with that.

In this case there seems to be a very clear connection between the use of the contraceptive drug and the symptoms, especially when we take the other circumstances into consideration, like age and lifestyle.

Too many people, who are taking prescription medication – or certain over the counter drugs for that matter – are not aware of what they are swallowing every day and what the side effects are. We should make it a rule to read up about whatever it is we put into our mouths, if it is something we never took before. There is so much information available out there and so easily accessible, that there really is no excuse anymore not to do that.

I have been working as a physiotherapist and acupuncturist for more than 30 years and after a while almost every condition that comes by I have already seen before. You develop a sixth sense for what might be wrong and what the treatment should be and if things don't add up an alarm bell rings. Every long-term health care practitioner can tell you that. That is why experience in these professions is so important. I have made it a rule to look up the side effects of medication my patients are using, when other options are a dead end and it always amazes me how often we can find a connection. Given the amount of drugs the average person is using these days, this is not a surprise. It also amazes me that the prescribers of these drugs don't tend to think in this direction. It is usually the patient himself who figures it out or another caregiver. Drugs are so much part of our existence that we take their working for granted and don't give it a second thought.

I remember this 14-year-old girl who had been complaining about her throat consistently. She had problems swallowing and had to clear her throat all the time. The family doctor referred her to a nose-ear-and throat specialist. He discovered that she still had her tonsils and that that probably was the problem. The parents wanted him to take them out, but he said that they were becoming more hesitant to do that when kids were older. He said that she could easily take antibiotics through her lifetime to suppress the infection. The parents did not accept that of course and tried to persuade the doctor to do the surgery. Eventually he decided to take them out and then the problem was solved. The recovery took maybe a little bit more time, but the alternative of having their young teenage daughter take antibiotics all the time was not acceptable for the parents and rightfully so. If a young person starts to take medication the body learns from an early stage that it does not have to work so hard to fix a problem, because it already had the experience of a drug that was doing the work. Bodies are lazy: if they don't have to they won't.

My 11-year-old daughter had shingles once. The doctor prescribed an (expensive) drug. The effects of drugs against shingles were slim in those days at the best. The pharmacist told me that I should not have high hopes and that he would probably not give those pills to his own daughter. We decided to leave the pills for what they were and two days later the shingles were gone and never came back.

We have to be our own doctor, especially when it comes to taking drugs. I have so many examples of people who have been taking prescription drugs for years and don't even know anymore if they are doing anything at all. Medication for acid reflux is a good example. I treated a lady who had been taking a prescription antacid for twenty years. I treated her with acupuncture and dietary advice. That dietary advice is available online and everyone can read it and see for himself if it makes sense.

After five treatments and a different diet her complaints were gone and she stopped taking her meds. The body had learned that it was supposed to do something about that acid reflux, because all of a sudden there were no more drugs.

Returning to the young woman with the swollen hands and feet. She was a little bit reluctant to try to change or stop her medication and that is understandable, because in her social environment almost all her female peers were doing the same, and many of them were not showing any symptoms, or maybe they did, but they contributed it to something else or just simply accepted it. Anyway, her complaints were almost gone after she stopped taking her medication.

Don't just take meds for granted, read the pamphlet and go online to get information. It is an obligation to our body.

Summary

These are just two examples. We should make it a rule to start questioning our self every time we experience a health issue. Most issues manifest themselves with some form of pain. Analyze the pain, the frequency, intensity and character of it. Remember that many pains are inflammation based and show swelling, redness and warmth and get worse with increased activity. If it is not inflammation then recognize the causing factors, changes in lifestyle, diet and behaviour. Many times the answers are not that far away.

Keep Eyes And Ears Open

Chapter 7

Learn And Apply

In a world where so many factors can threaten our health and where we can read all the time about the dangers of heart attacks, high blood pressure, diabetes and strokes, it is understandable that we don't want to run the risk of missing something. On the other hand, all this information and possible risks are feeding our fear and fear is one of the strongest factors to make us sick. So, we have to find a way to balance between the two. We don't want to miss out, but we also don't want to be afraid of everything. This is not so easy. We can go for regular medical check-ups. That might ease our minds, if the results of the tests are negative. But what if something comes back positive? There can always be something positive, do we really need to know that? Take the screening for breast cancer for example. Recent Canadian research has shown that annual mammograms often do more harm than good, because they over-diagnose many breast cancers that are actually harmless. In the meantime women are worried and stressed and stress helps with the formation of cancer cells. The same seems to be true for screening of prostate cancer. We don't always need to know everything that goes on in our body. In fact more and more studies show that a relaxed state of mind, meditation and confidence in one's own healing system is the best medication for almost everything. Stress shows itself mainly through symptoms of tiredness, depression, anxiety, insomnia, high blood pressure, headache, skin diseases etc., but eventually long-term exposure to stress will affect our total health. A human being cannot always be tired, because it means that it is lacking energy and therefore it does not have the power to fight any intruders and sickness will spread. This concept of energy was already part of ancient thinking.

If we want to find a middle way between fear and missing out, a good way is to monitor our state of health continuously. We all have built-in warning signs that tell us if something really bad is going on and if going to a doctor is imminent. But if we don't feel like that, and a complaint persists and really bothers us, we need to decide whether we want to see a doctor. The doctor will do his own diagnosis and either prescribe medication, give advice or refer to a different discipline. Regardless of what happens, this is the time to learn. Most of the time the issue that we are seeking help for represents a weakness in our system, meaning that it might be a recurring thing. If we have weak sinuses for example, we will probably have weak sinuses for the rest of our life. We don't want to visit the doctor all the time because we have a sinus problem. Suppose the doctor finds a chronic sinus infection and prescribes an anti inflammatory like corticosteroids. The first time that happens, we will take the medication and experience the effects it has on our complaints. If the complaints go away, we will probably go back for more the next time the sinuses act up. Our body has learned that there is something out there that can fix the problem. So it more or less expects the same thing to happen the next time. If we don't want this passive approach, but we want to be more involved in the healing process, we'll have to teach our body that there are also other ways, maybe not so fast working as the corticosteroids, but milder and more balanced. The sinus infection is obviously an inflammation, something our whole body has to deal with all the time. Inflammation tends to go to sinuses because it is a confined space with only a small way out, so an ideal location for infection. What we want to do is bring the chance of inflammation down. We have already seen that there are many ways of doing that, starting with our food intake. We can decide to follow an anti inflammatory diet, drink lots of water to flush the mucus out, rinse our nose and sinuses with a salty water solution and drink less coffee and alcohol, because they can increase the inflammation. We can also decide to rest more and meditate, two natural ways of fighting inflammation. There are also many herbal and natural remedies against inflammation. Acupuncture is a very good alternative treatment solution, in combination with the suggestions made above.

Our body will also learn from this experience. It will learn that it possesses a lot of options to fight the inflammation and that it can produce its own anti-inflammatory chemicals.

Now it is a matter of what we offer our body most. If we keep taking the corticosteroids our body will become less and less sensitive for an alternative solution and in the end only the drugs will work. But over time we need to take more and more to get any effect.

We have learned after this experience how our body reacts on the different treatment methods and we have seen that we can apply homemade treatments that are effective, maybe not so fast, but more stabile overtime. The more we apply this the more sensitive our body becomes for mild homemade approaches. The next time, we might not have to see the doctor.

This might sound like a very simple and logical solution, but in reality it does not work like that. The majority of the people with a chronic sinus infection visit the doctor every time there is a flare up. And there will be flare-ups, because they don't make any changes in their approach of the problem.

Let's talk about a 22-year-old female student, who is active in sports, but who experiences shoulder pain and pain in the foot every time she sports, walks or runs. Intake and assessment show no loss of strength and no limited range of motion. She is not overweight, sleeps well and has a healthy appetite. She is bright and generally a happy person, who knows what she wants.

The complaints have been there since she started being active in sports. At first sight there is not much that would explain her complaints. Then I ask her to make some general movements with her shoulders and I see immediately that she has a larger range of motion than would be normal for a woman her age. It means that she is hypermobile, a condition that is often seen in young women. Flexibility of the ligaments that surround a joint determine the stability and range of motion of that joint. If the ligaments are loose and flexible they allow more movement and cannot protect the joint properly. It is now up to the muscles to guide and move the joint and take over some of the protection. But muscles are not built for that. They are built to move and when they get tired they cannot protect anymore and the joint starts to hurt. Because this young woman was very active in sports, she used her muscles a lot and eventually developed a chronic pain in her joints. The shoulder joint is especially sensitive to this, because it is the most movable joint we have, with an almost 360 degrees range.

The foot is also sensitive, because the ligaments have to support the arch of the foot. If the ligaments are weak, all the jumping and landing and sprinting become too much and a chronic pain can develop.

The solution for this problem is twofold. First of all the patient must understand what is going on. If not, the problem will come back again and again. The next thing is to strengthen the muscles around the joint to provide as much support as possible. She has to spend a lot of time doing exercises if she wants to stay as active as she is now. And even then she will be limited, because the muscles cannot fully take over from ligaments and joint capsule.

The pain someone experiences from hypermobility is typical. It is a ligament pain, so it usually is better during controlled movement, but worse when resting or sleeping, when the mass of the body hangs in the ligaments without protection of the muscles.

Eventually ligament pain can become very bad. In the Middle Ages they used to hang people bound by the wrists from a high beam and just let them hang. The first half hour or so the muscles would be able to compensate and take the weight away from the joints and ligaments, but after that, when the muscles were tired and needed oxygen, the result was an agonizing pain; very devious and very effective.

What this young woman has learned is that her body reacts that way when she is very active in sports or any other strenuous physical activity, or when she makes repetitive movements, like lifting or carrying. She will recognize the typical pain and she will know what is going on. She can then do what she knows will help her. She also has learned that medication will not solve the problem.

She has been her own doctor after having learned what was going on the first time.

Summary

We can only learn if we keep our eyes and ears open. If we do that, we will recognize signs and symptoms and we can supply a solution that we know works, because it worked before. This will make us more confident and less preoccupied with our problem.

There Is A Certain Comfort In Being Sick

Chapter 8

Being Our Own Doctor Is Not For Everyone

Many people simply do not know the mechanisms that make them sick and therefore they also lack the ability to get better. They first have to understand. It is a learning process that has to be stimulated by others and by trial and error.

There is definitely a big change going on in the way people perceive health. They are trying to own it more, compared to earlier times when our health was the doctor's problem. But there are still many people who don't want to become involved. Most of these non-committers are older, being raised in those times when the doctor was part of the important people like the lawyer and the notary and they simply followed their directions. Many of these older people now need more medical attention, because they have a less active lifestyle and don't like making changes.

These patients keep filling up the waiting rooms of doctor's offices and hospitals and are not really involved in trying to be their own doctor. I still remember one of my first patients after my graduation for physiotherapy in the Netherlands. I was enthusiastically explaining what he could do himself at home to improve his condition. At a certain point he asked, literally: "Is there no pill for that?" As a just starting professional I was shocked that somebody could think like that.

Another sign that people not always want to be involved in their own health care process is that they don't want to do exercises. In physiotherapy doing exercises is the most important modality of the treatment and without that most people do not get better. I always give exercises, regardless of the problem. Even if patients come in with a headache or complaints about tiredness they need to do exercises, if only to involve them in the process. They always say yes, but if their condition does not get better, I know they don't. Understanding the mechanisms that make us sick opens up a wide view and perspective, not only about health, but also about life itself. Life makes us sick, if we don't try to live it in a responsible way. It is not so difficult to try to live life in a responsible way and a lot of rules and regulations come automatically.

People only do well when they socialize and communicate with others. They are supposed to respect others and get respect back, but if they live only for themselves they eventually will get sick. Our nervous system is being fed by positive attention from others, like appreciation, respect, compliments, admiration and stimulation. People get sick when they are alone and when their basic needs are not fulfilled. They become depressed and lose energy and cannot fight anymore.

The more we are focused on our self, the more chance we have to get sick. And we are living in a time of self, where the ego comes first. No wonder there is so much sickness, depression and misery. Being concentrated only on our self is not very clever.

Not only is being our own doctor not for everyone, it is also true that not everyone wants to get better. **There is a certain comfort in being sick.** It can be a reason to be excused of certain activities that we don't like. It can also be used to manipulate others to do what we want them to do. Above all, being sick is a great way of getting attention, something we all want. And once we have that, we don't easily want to give it up. I remember the lady who was suffering from migraine headaches for more than 25 years. She had done all kinds of treatments, but nothing really worked. Finally she decided to do a relaxation therapy and de-stressing. Her headaches were as good as gone once she mastered that. She went home happy, but after a few months she came back. When we asked if her headache came back she said no, but the fact that she could not use her headache anymore as an excuse in her daily life was something she could not handle. It brought tension in her marriage, because she could not say no anymore if her husband wanted her to go to a party or a visit. She actually asked if we could bring at least some of the headache back, so that she would have part of her life back!

Another nice example about not wanting to lose certain unhealthy habits is this one. When I started acupuncture in the Netherlands, we had a patient in our university clinic that wanted to quit smoking. He was 70 years old, smoked two packs a day since he was 15 and drank about 8 glasses of brandy per day. We gave him a general treatment against addiction and one week later he came back. He said he was still smoking, but he did not like his drinks anymore! He found that very inconvenient, because he did not want to quit drinking in his social life, but he wanted to lose the cigarettes. Unfortunately the body does not choose between addictions, so he had to accept the situation.

A person does not develop a chronic physical illness just like that. Almost everybody with chronic pain, for example, also has a chronic mental issue. That can be anything, like an unhappy relationship, or a very dissatisfying work situation, or not being happy with one self. Many times people don't really want the confrontation with them selves, so they accept the situation and suffer the physical pain. It is clear that by being our own doctor and by trying to solve the problems in the background, we can make quite a difference in the physical problems we experience. But sometimes it is hard to make changes and we choose for the status quo. As I said being our own doctor is not for everyone.

Summary

Some people don't want to be their own doctor, because they firmly believe that they miss the knowledge. Others cherish the benefits of being sick, because it plays an important role in their social life. There is a certain comfort in being sick, most of all because it gives us attention.

**Most Patients Don't Expect To Get
What They Deserve**

Chapter 9

The Way It Should Be

A couple of times already I have mentioned the business aspect of health. We all know that at the end of the day money is more important than health in the eyes of people who make their living off somebody else's health.

In the beginning I could hardly believe it. I always assumed that all our noses would point in the same direction and that we all wanted the best medication, for a reasonable price as soon as possible. How naïve could I be.

I am not going to write a long story about the bad sales promoting techniques of pharmaceutical companies, because we all know that already. Besides, it is a very vague and difficult area for people who are not immediately involved and absolutely not transparent. It is enough to know that when we enter a doctor's office and leave with a prescription, that particular drug is most likely the result of an interaction between the physician and a representative of a pharmaceutical company, who did his best, to be as persuasive as possible. We can read about big companies who are implementing new transparent rules for their reps, how to approach a prescriber and be as open and clear as possible, but in the end, all they want is to sell their products, the more the better. So a new giftwrap does not make a lot of difference.

And because it is such a vague and in-transparent business, it is even more important to try to stay away from medication and drugs, by living a healthy lifestyle.

I happen to have a good relationship with my GP. He is clear, knowledgeable and willing to listen to what I want. He is not a high prescriber; at least that is what I want to believe. He sometimes prescribes a drug, just because he is involved with my problem and he wants to help. So he might prescribe a drug, because he heard that some people had good results with it. He basically puts the ball in my corner, and that is where it belongs. It is then up to me to read about it and see if I want to take it. Most of the time I don't, but at least there was a healthy interaction between us. Although it is of the utmost importance to be fully involved with our own disease and its possible solutions, it is just as important that a doctor is looking at our problem the same way. He needs to be fully involved with our problem, because he is a doctor and he wants to have a good night sleep after a day of work. He wants to have the feeling that he did a good job and that he tried to help his patients to the best of his abilities and that is not the same as prescribing medication.

Health care practitioners should be completely focused on the matter at hand and I know how difficult that can be. On a normal day I see about 20 patients and they all have a complicated life story and they all deserve my attention. After years of practice it can sometimes become a bit of a chore to listen every day and find solutions. Sometimes I want to tell my own story and I want my patients to listen, but I know that is the worst thing a practitioner can do. We are there to listen, not the other way around.

Sometimes, I feel guilty, because I have not given a patient my complete attention for whatever reason. It can be so bad, that I decide to call the patient and ask about his wellbeing and offer my apologies. Many times they don't even know what I am talking about. And that is a bad thing, **because they already expect not to get what they deserve.** That attitude is what makes doctors and other health care professionals cocky. They assume that the patient will accept whatever they say and it seems that the higher we get on the medical professional ladder, the worse it gets. Medical specialists are at the top of the chain. Their expertise is too complicated for many users to grasp and they don't have anybody to respond to. So basically, they can do what they want. They don't expect a lot of arguments against their opinion and when they get some it usually ends in a very tense doctor/patient relationship and that is never in our advantage. Still, there are general rules of respect and human interaction. Waiting for half an hour or more in a waiting room, while being perfectly on time for the appointment, and then being directed and prepared by a nurse to be ready for the attack on our integrity by a person who does not apologize and sometimes does not introduce himself is quite unacceptable. Our time is just as valuable as his and, most importantly, he makes his money because of people like us.

Thankfully, I don't have many of those encounters, because if I did, I don't think I would survive long, being the underdog in a battle against a guy with a knife.

How can we get better, when we have an experience like that? All it does is raising our stress level, preparing our body for a flight, fight and fear reaction, becoming defensive, soaking in adrenaline and cortisol, all the while being involved in a procedure that is supposed to be beneficial to our health.

It is baffling, but it is also a daily truth for many patients. It is even worse for people who are less assertive and more trusting. They are overwhelmed and go home, thinking that from now on everything will get better. They can have a hard time interpreting the signs of their body and just go to another confrontation if they don't feel better. Maybe, if we think about it, being one hundred percent trusting and accepting and believing is the best thing to do, because then the mind guides us to healing. It all depends on the person, but I am sure that the majority of the readers will agree that a respectful and individual approach works best.

Wanting to be our own doctor and at the same time having to visit a doctor can sometimes be challenging, for both parties. On the other hand I am a firm believer in cooperation. The only goal for both the practitioner and the patient is to get the patient better. However that is achieved is unimportant. If patient and doctor can do that together it is even more rewarding. If either the patient's or the doctor's ego gets in the way there are two losers. That is one of the reasons why I believe that being a physiotherapist can be more rewarding than being a medical doctor, because the main value of physiotherapy is practise and exercise and only the patient himself can do that.

Summary

Pharmaceutical companies are often more interested in the sale of their products than the eventual healing of the disease. Only the patient himself can be fully unbiased about his problems in search for a real solution. The relationship between health care practitioner and patient should be one of mutual respect and the patient is entitled to complete attention for his problems. The only goal for practitioner and patient is to get the patient better and however that is achieved is unimportant. A well-prepared patient can engage in a useful discussion with the practitioner and find the best solution.

A Hospital Should Have A Customer Service Desk Instead Of An Admission Desk

Chapter 10

Respect – We Are First And For All Customers

At the moment the business of health care is in the hands of others than us. It is a huge business, with billions of dollars involved, that we, patients and taxpayers, are paying for. Because it is so close to our wellbeing and can be so complicated, we are very insecure when it comes to making decisions. The industry uses that to its advantage. It uses our insecurity to make money. Something like that, when it happens to others, infuriates us, and we say 'I would never allow that', but in the end we all put our fate in the hands of the same institution.

Health is not the only thing that is close to our wellbeing. What about money? Without money there is not much wellbeing. When it comes to investing for our future, we might hire a professional, but we keep a very close look at the process and what is going to happen with our dollars. Everybody accepts that and encourages that, even the hired professionals.

What about buying a house, a very important part of our wellbeing. We hire a real estate agent, because he has access to resources that can help us selling or buying a house quicker. But we are totally involved in the process and we don't leave everything in the hands of the realtor. Eventually it is us who make the end decision.

What about getting married and having children? Those are all major and very emotional decisions. But isn't our health also a very emotional asset?

Nobody has anything to do with our decision to get married and whether or not to have children. But the decision is emotionally charged and very complicated and determines the rest of our lives. Exactly the same as decisions about our health can be.

So why are we so lenient when it comes to decisions about our health? Is it because it is complicated? Maybe, but that is why we have health care professionals that we can turn to and ask for advice. Just like we can ask the realtor or the investments broker. But the decision and initiative should be ours and we should be critical and demand explanation and respect.

When we can treat health care the same as we treat any other business that wants our dollars, then we become customers in stead of patients and customers always come first. Instead of going to a hospital and being treated like a number, we now go to the customer service department and are treated as the most important asset of the business. Without us there is no job, no money, please don't forget that.

When we are suffering from a lot of health issues and need more doctor and hospital care, it becomes a habit to just follow whatever anybody tells us and the more subdued we become, the bolder the other party becomes. That is human nature, we like to dominate and wield power. But especially then should we demand respect and not be afraid to say what we think.

I remember my mother-in-law, whom I accompanied to a visit to a doctor in the hospital. It was about her carpal tunnel syndrome and the doctor ordered her, while looking into some paperwork, absentmindedly, to take her clothes off and lie down on the table! What do you mean, respect?

We have to stop behaving like underdogs and demand attention and being listened to. Stop being patient. We are customers and not subjects that can be pushed around. Our health is an important asset that people want to service, so give us the same attention we get when we bring our car for service. Don't forget, it is our health.

Summary

Too often patients, paying customers, are not treated with the respect they deserve, assuming they probably have no idea what it is all about. We should no longer accept that and show that we can be prepared and can ask useful questions that help us in our decision to undergo medical care.

Be Open To The Magic Around Us

Chapter 11

Guidelines

So, you have read my book and now you are all hyper and demand respect and immediately want to take control over your own health. How are you going to do that? Is there a schedule?

Well first of all I hope that I have awakened your feeling of self-awareness and self-respect. It goes without saying that, when demanding respect, you need to give respect. So don't go running to the first available health care professional and start shouting at him, that you don't accept it any longer, because I assure you that will not work.

Being aware of yourself and feeling your own value will automatically guide you in the process of demanding respect. There is one little glitch here. As I said before, this is a time of self. The concept of self is extremely exaggerated, as everyone is trying to portrait himself as a combination of a Hollywood star, nobleman and employee-of-the-month. Just take a look at social media and you will drown in them. That is not the feeling of self-value I mean. That kind of exposure is cheap, volatile and empty. What I mean is that every human being has value, wherever he comes from or whatever he does. Just nurture that value and be sure of yourself and people will automatically treat you in a different way. You'll get a smile when you smile.

Suppose you are developing a health issue, let's say a headache. It is very important to trace back when and how your headache started, because you want to know the circumstances in your life at that time. Is it the first time you experience this headache? What were you dong when it started, did it come on slowly or acute? Do you remember if you were experiencing stress at that time? Did you change your diet recently? Did you change your job or were you making repetitive movements that were tiring you? Don't forget that a stressful period you went through months ago can easily now translate itself in a headache or any other symptom for that matter, even when the actual stressor does not exist anymore. The body needs time to adjust and will have to deal sooner or later with the effects the stress caused.

After you have eliminated all possible factors that might have caused your headache, Tylenol does not work and you still don't see any rhyme or reason, you might want to consider visiting a doctor, physiotherapist or chiropractor or whomever you feel comfortable with. Be sure when you go there that you know what you want to talk about, what kind of questions you want to ask and what you want the practitioner to do for you. Be prepared to give your opinion about possible things that he might suggest, especially, when you visit an MD, when he wants you to do blood work or make an X-ray. Be very critical when you visit a chiropractor about having taken all those X-rays. It is always better in a case like this, to first do the things that have less impact on your physical integrity. For example, doing exercises to improve your posture and strengthen muscles, has less impact than a chiropractic adjustment, and is also an activity that you do yourself. If that does not work, an adjustment might be indicated (with or without an X-ray), if you are a person who is into adjustments. Adjustments are not for everybody; as a matter of fact nothing is for everybody. If you finally end up with the MD, you can tell him what you already did and what worked and what not. Now the decision to do blood work or take an X-ray is easier to make and to understand and there is less chance that public dollars are spent on something that might lead to nothing. Don't forget whom you are visiting, the doctor wants to doctor, the surgeon wants to surgeon, the chiropractor wants to chiropractor and the physio wants to physio. And they all have very convincing arguments why you should follow their advice. So you have to be prepared and as knowledgeable as possible, but that is ok, because you have to fight for yourself and protect your integrity.

Weigh all the possibilities and discuss them with your doctor. If he does not want to go that route or if he does not like critical patients, find another doctor. The relationship between you and your health care practitioner is very important and should not get in the way of your choice to be your own doctor. What is right for one is not right for another. I am very satisfied with my doctor, but I recently spoke with a patient who had left him, because they couldn't go through the same door together.

That can happen.

Try to find out in every way you can what might be wrong with you. Talk to people, not just professionals and find out what they think or what kind of experience they had.

Follow the lead that you feel comfortable with. There is no written truth in any case. The way I am treating my patients is based on my views and what I think is important, but that might not be the same way my patient thinks. Even if my patient chooses a way that is against my views, but he feels comfortable with it, chances are he will heal faster than if he would have followed my advice.

I have treated a lot of Europeans and North Americans in the past. They all have their own special things and issues, but a noticeable difference is that in North America people tend to take more medication and are more open to surgery. I once read an article called The American Syndrome. It was about (North) Americans over 60 years old. The majority of them would be taking medication for cholesterol, high blood pressure, thyroid imbalance, diabetes type 2 and acid reflux. Many of them would be taking that for years, adding a lot of toxic material to their bodies in the process. At the moment I am treating a patient who has been doing exactly that. He is complaining about lower back pain in combination with acid reflux. When the acid reflux becomes worse his back pain gets worse. I am treating him with acupuncture and there is some progress after a few treatments. I told him to rethink the amount of drugs he is taking. His doctor thinks that some of them could cause the acidity and they tried already to reduce it a bit, but he is still taking a lot of medication.

There is a fair chance that his complaints will be a lot more manageable if he can get himself to reduce most of his drugs, with or without help from his doctor. But I can feel in his reactions that he is not ready for that and does not totally support the idea. So what is wisdom in this case? I am sure that it will help him, because I have seen it happen many times. The use of drugs is not written in stone and we should be critical about it. Having been diagnosed with diabetes type 2 does not automatically mean that you have to take drugs for the rest of your life. The same goes for high blood pressure and many other diagnoses. But what if the patient believes the drugs are necessary and he cannot do without? Then it might be advisable for him to keep taking it and in the meantime figure out what would be the best approach for his problems. The power of the mind should not be underestimated. Anyway, whatever happens, the most important thing is that the patient starts thinking about his situation and is becoming critical. Now he can ask purposeful questions and try to find a way that is comfortable for him.

We also have to learn to trust our instincts. Most truth is in our instincts and we don't need scientific proof of everything we try to decide. I just read about a scientific study that found that if people meet and are romantically interested in each other they tend to look at the eyes, but if they are more sexually interested in each other they look more at the rest of the body. Wow, I am so glad that that has now been scientifically established; it really has so much influence on my future behaviour and, honestly, I had no idea!

Sometimes we forget that we are just people and behave like people and that we don't need a certificate to make a cup of coffee or pick our nose.

After having been critical and gathering knowledge and after having tried some different approaches it is time to look at your own lifestyle. Everybody knows exactly what he does wrong and what he should improve, regardless of what the media say and what is fashionable. We know if we eat the right things, if we are active enough and whether or not we are spending enough time on relaxation and de-stressing.

We all are fighting our own little battle with these things. Just don't go over the top. Look at the hype about weight loss. I am very much aware of the fact that the world is suffering from a huge amount of overweight and obese people and that it is a serious health problem. But the solutions that are offered are often not any healthier. Any given day you can find at least 10 new ways of losing 8 pounds per week if you just read enough magazines. You know what I mean, those magazines that only need two words on their cover to sell: sex and weight loss.

These kinds of diets are not giving any long-term solution, are not healthy and are definitely not in balance with the body. As I said before, everything in the body goes slow and needs time to adjust and suddenly cutting out all sugars, carbohydrates or fats after years of overeating, is not my idea of balance. We are not all looking like models and that is also absolutely unimportant. What we need to do is consult with ourselves and find out what needs to be changed and do it slowly. Slow and responsible weight loss is always more satisfactory and lasting than just another diet. The same goes for physical activity and relaxation. Going to a gym every day, after years of not going at all, is out of balance and our body will let us know. If we have never tried to relax and all of a sudden we are lying on the floor for hours and read everything there is about yoga and transcendental meditation, we will not succeed and we will become frustrated. It is ok to skip a day, or two, just as it is ok to eat cake or cookies when there is a birthday, as long as we are consistent and, last but not least, as long as we believe in what we are doing. Remember, it is all about individuality, finding our own way. We can immediately recognize somebody who has decided to make some changes and is serious about it. Their behaviour has changed and they are more self assured and consistent.

Another point of advice is to keep it simple. We have a tendency to drown in all our new ideas and we want to do everything at the same time. If you decided to make changes, then go step by step. First work on your diet, that is complicated enough in the beginning. Give your body the chance to get used to the new regime. Bodies get used to almost everything if you just give them time. If you eat 4000 calories every day your body thinks that that is the norm and will expect all 4000 of them. If you –slowly- start reducing your calorie intake and are at 3500 after two weeks, your body will think that that is the norm and so on. It will not ask anymore for the other 500 calories, because it has forgotten about them. If you want to go down with medication that you take every day, don't start by taking them every other day, because that is a 50% reduction and your body will be confused and ask for more, frustrating you. Try 10% per week for example and wait if you can see any changes before you go to the next batch. Try to substitute what you take less with good food, like fruits or vegetables, or maybe some herbal medication.

Once you have your diet change under control and you feel comfortable about it and don't have to force yourself every time, you are ready for the next step.

Slowly introduce more physical activity into your life. If you don't want to visit a gym and sweat with the body builders, which can be overwhelming, I'll tell you, there are many things you can do yourself at home or outside. Walking, cycling, jogging, floor exercises on a mat or on a big exercise ball, using free weights etc. Do that until you feel comfortable enough to go to a gym and become more serious. A gym, despite the steroid addicts, can be a stimulating and motivating place and help you in your endeavours. Now you have been changing your diet and preparing your body to be happy with less and healthier food and that makes you feel better already and stimulates you to improve your performance in the gym. These two things go together, because our bodies like to be healthy and in balance and when the right ingredients are there they will only cooperate. The body and the mind don't want to be out of balance, it is us that force them to it.

With a healthy diet and enough physical activity we have been preparing our body to start some relaxation. That is a reward and should always be done after the other two. During my time on cruise ships I saw how well that was set up by the cruise companies. There were lots of healthy food choices, if one wanted, huge gyms and physical activity classes and plenty of opportunity to relax afterwards in a sauna, on a deck chair or during a yoga class. When the body is well fed and nicely circulated it is more than ready to relax and the best time to learn meditation is then.

All these activities help our brain produce a wave of endorphins and other feel good hormones and that is what makes us want to go again. Slowly we manoeuvre our body and mind into a new regimen, one that we like, that the body likes and feels comfortable with. Once we have experienced this feeling of wellbeing, it becomes an addiction in itself, but this time a good addiction, one that we are allowed to succumb to. It is difficult to go back to an unhealthy lifestyle afterwards. Besides, an unhealthy lifestyle is associated with other negative circumstances, like lots of stress, expectations, junk food, smoking and physical inactivity. It is all up to you if you want to go back there, but you have seen that it can be different.

I talked before about the concept of what I call magic. **If you want to be a successful self-doctor you have to be open to the magic around you.** The reason is that magic carries so much healing in it, that it would be such a waste not to use it.

Magic is everywhere. It is of course visible in the different forms of nature around you, whether you live in a city or somewhere rural. It is enjoying a sunset or an approaching thunderstorm or one of these amazing big moons we can see in the summer. Living in North America can be mesmerizing in that respect, especially coming from Europe. Every day I am enjoying these amazing skies and weather systems I can see here, from blizzards to rainbows and from cloud formations to rain showers. Living here makes being in contact with magic a lot easier. Of course magic is not just nature, but just about everything that thrills us and amazes us. Magic can be a good conversation with a total stranger or a glass of wine while reading a good book. But it can also be a walk with your grandson or winning $5 in the lottery. It can be seeing a smile on somebody's face or listening to good music. Whatever it is for you is not important. Important is that it happens everyday and that you open up for it everyday.

Being aware of magic makes you feel good and automatically brings body and mind in balance and then you are already healing yourself right there. It is not so complicated once you have decided to open your eyes.

Magic is important because it appeals to our basic needs. Our basic needs are also simple. We want to be appreciated and loved and we want to be recognised for what we are. And most of all we want to feel good. If we can invent something that makes people feel good we will all be millionaires, guaranteed.

We are humans and therefore social beings. As long as we can live together we can fulfill our basic needs. How can we be appreciated and loved if we are alone? That is not going to happen. Unfortunately, this is the time where people are trying desperately to be noticed, but because there are so many of us it is almost impossible to get the attention we need. As a result many become depressed and isolate them selves. If nobody gives us attention, the least we can do is give attention to our self. I am not a psychologist, but for me, that is the reason for all those tattoos, earphones and focusing on cellphones and even for all those weirdoes running around with guns: the ultimate form of attracting attention.

If we cannot get other peoples attention in the usual way, we should try to become comfortable with our self and with our qualities and accomplishments and spread that around. That will get attention. That will bring us more in balance: another advantage of being our own doctor.

Being our own doctor makes us feel good. We get addicted to good feelings; therefore we become addicted to being our own doctor. There are worse things to get addicted to.

Summary

Being aware of your self and your value will help you getting respect. Be prepared to discuss your problems with the doctor and have the facts lined up. Choose the way of treating that appeals most to you, whatever it is, even choosing for medication.
Trust your instincts and monitor your lifestyle to find out where it went wrong. Choose a smart solution and don't overdo it. Overdoing never leads to something good. Make a program that is simple to fulfil.
By being comfortable with our self and our qualities and accomplishments, we can keep depression away and give attention to our self.

Conclusion

Everything around us is changing. Things are not what they were anymore, even after just a couple of years. What we took for granted in the past might not have any value right now. That happens everywhere and definitely also in the way we look at healthcare. Studying and learning used to be something for the happy few, an elite group of people in society, who passed it on from generation to generation. There used to be a time where tradespeople were seen as lowly educated people, with not much perspective and now a good carpenter can make almost as much as a lawyer or a psychologist. People are more aware of their value in society and they are better informed. Everybody with a computer can read up just about everything and form an opinion about it. We have become critical and demanding consumers and the business world is reacting accordingly. They cater to the customer's every whim.

This is the way it should be. If they want our money, they have to deliver a good product in a pleasant and professional way.

In healthcare things are a little bit different. Patients are often seen as laymen about the details of their problem and are assumed to follow orders. Many people comply and when that happens we automatically hand control to the experts and go with the flow. In my opinion, that is never a good thing to do, whatever the circumstances. Giving away control is feeding the ego of the other and is the same as handing over power. When we hand over power, the other person will eventually always do what is best for him and not so much what is best for us. That is the way humans work. **We need to interact with each other in order to establish a mutually beneficial relationship.** We do this in almost every possible situation, for example when we buy consumer goods, or when we have a conversation with somebody or request somebodies help. But it always stops with healthcare. It is like we are afraid to know something about our health, to have an opinion about it. People immediately become insecure and uncertain, when their health is involved. Sometimes that is understandable, when the situation is grave and threatening, but many times it is not, but we still surrender fully. That creates an unhealthy situation. It puts a lot of responsibility and expectation on the shoulder of the practitioner, where it really does not belong and it makes the patient lazy and inert. And often, when something goes wrong, the patient blames the practitioner for not doing his job right. That is the easy way out, but the system allows it.

We need to change the system, starting with our self. Apply the same self-assuredness to our health as we do to everything else. That requires knowledge of course, but if we can acquire knowledge about cars and computers we want to buy, we can also do that for our health situation. Only us, the patients, can make this happen. As long as we keep passing the control to somebody else, nothing will change and we will be pushed around forever.

It is time to wake up and show our self and the world who we are and what we want, both in the showroom and in the treatment room. After some initial resistance it will only be appreciated, make healthcare cheaper and boost our self-esteem.